ABC OF

SPINAL CORD INJURY

Second edition

ABC OF

SPINAL CORD INJURY

SECOND EDITION

DAVID GRUNDY FRCS
*Consultant in spinal injuries, Duke of Cornwall Spinal Treatment Centre,
Odstock Hospital, Salisbury*

ANDREW SWAIN FRCS
*Consultant in accident and emergency medicine
General Hospital, Weston-super-Mare*

with contributions from

ERICA BAMFORD, JOHN CUMMING, HILARY DOVER,
JANE HENSHAW, ANTHONY TROMANS, TRUDY WARD, CATRIONA WOOD

Published by the BMJ Publishing Group
Tavistock Square, London WC1H 9JR

First published 1986
Reprinted 1989
Reprinted 1990
Reprinted 1991

Second edition 1993

British Library Cataloguing in Publication Data
Grundy, David
  ABC of Spinal Cord Injury. – 2 Rev. ed
  I. Title II. Swain, Andrew
617.4

ISBN 0-7279-0760-3

The photograph on page 1 is taken from:
Hughes J T. The Edwin Smith Papyrus.
Paraplegia 1988; 26: 71–82

Printed in Great Britain at the University Press, Cambridge
Typesetting by Apek Typesetters, Avon House, Blackfriars Road,
Nailsea, Bristol BS19 2DJ

Contents

	Page
At the accident A SWAIN, D GRUNDY	1
Evacuation and initial management at hospital A SWAIN, D GRUNDY	4
Radiological investigations D GRUNDY, A SWAIN	7
Early management and complications—I D GRUNDY, A SWAIN	12
Early management and complications—II D GRUNDY, A SWAIN	16
Medical management in the spinal injuries unit D GRUNDY, ANTHONY TROMANS, *consultant in spinal injuries, Duke of Cornwall Spinal Treatment Centre*	19
Urological management D GRUNDY, JOHN CUMMING, *consultant urologist, Southampton University Hospitals and Duke of Cornwall Spinal Treatment Centre*	24
Nursing CATRIONA WOOD, *nurse teacher, Duke of Cornwall Spinal Treatment Centre,* D GRUNDY	30
Physiotherapy TRUDY WARD, *superintendent physiotherapist, Duke of Cornwall Spinal Treatment Centre,* D GRUNDY	36
Occupational therapy JANE HENSHAW, *head occupational therapist, Duke of Cornwall Spinal Treatment Centre,* D GRUNDY	40
Social needs of patient and family ERICA BAMFORD, *senior social worker, Duke of Cornwall Spinal Treatment Centre,* D GRUNDY	43
Transfer of care from hospital to community HILARY DOVER, *community liaison nurse, Duke of Cornwall Spinal Treatment Centre,* D GRUNDY	46
Later management and complications—I D GRUNDY, A TROMANS	50
Later management and complications—II D GRUNDY, A TROMANS	54
Index	57

AT THE ACCIDENT

Andrew Swain, David Grundy

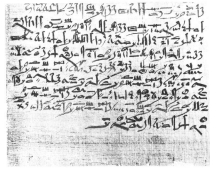

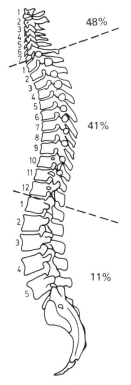

48%

41%

11%

Spinal cord injury is a mortal condition and has been recognised as such since antiquity. In about 2500 BC, in the Edwin Smith papyrus, an unknown Egyptian physician accurately described the clinical features of traumatic tetraplegia (quadriplegia) and revealed an awareness of the awful prognosis with the chilling advice: "an ailment not to be treated." That view prevailed until the early years of this century. In the first world war 90% of patients who suffered a spinal cord injury died within one year of wounding and only about 1% survived more than 20 years. Fortunately, the vision of a few pioneers—Guttmann in the United Kingdom together with Munro and Bors in the United States—has greatly improved the outlook for those with spinal cord injury, although the mortality associated with tetraplegia was still 35% in the 1960s. The better understanding and management of spinal cord injury have led to a reduction in mortality and a higher incidence of incomplete spinal cord damage in those who survive. Ideal management now demands immediate evacuation from the scene of the accident to a centre where intensive care of the patient can be supervised by a specialist in spinal cord injuries.

At present the annual incidence of spinal cord injury within the United Kingdom is about 10 to 15 per million of the population. In recent years there has been an increase in the proportion of injuries to the cervical spinal cord and this is now the most common indication for admission to a spinal injuries unit.

Although the effect of the initial trauma is irreversible, the spinal cord is at risk from further injury by injudicious early management. The emergency services must avoid such complications, in unconscious patients by being aware of the possibility of spinal cord injury from the nature of the accident and in conscious patients by suspecting the diagnosis from the history and basic neurological assessment. If such an injury is suspected the patient may be handled correctly from the outset.

Causes of spinal cord injury—New patient admissions to Duke of Cornwall Spinal Treatment Centre, 1989-91					
Road traffic accidents	51·5%	Domestic and Industrial accidents	27%	Injuries at sport	16%
Car, van, or lorry	27%	Domestic—eg falls down stairs		Diving into shallow water	7%
Motorcycle	21%	or from trees or ladders	16%	Rugby	2·5%
Cycle	2·5%	Accidents at work—eg falls		Horse riding	1%
Pedestrian	1%	from scaffolding or ladders,		Miscellaneous—gymnastics,	
		crush injuries	11%	Motocross, skiing, parachuting,	
				etc.	5·5%
Self harm and criminal assault	5%	Major incident			
Self harm	4·5%	Air crash	0·5%		
Criminal assault	0·5%				

Management at the scene of the accident

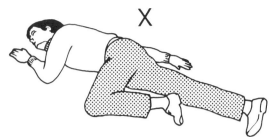

Standard recovery position—note that the spine is rotated.

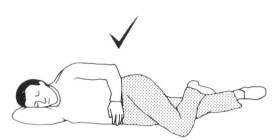

Stable lateral position, avoiding spinal rotation.

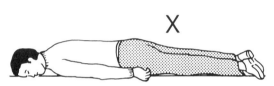

Prone position compromises respiration.

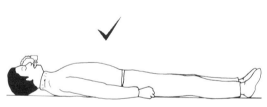

If patient is supine the airway must be protected fully.

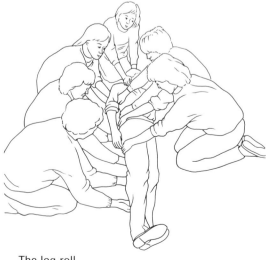

The log roll.

Doctors may witness or attend the scene of an accident, particularly if the casualty is trapped. After release there may be anxieties about moving patients if they complain of pain in the back or neck, describe altered sensation or loss of power in the limbs, or are unconscious.

The unconscious patient

It must be assumed that the force that rendered the patient unconscious has injured the cervical spine until radiography of its entire length proves otherwise. Until then the head and neck must be carefully placed and held in the neutral (anatomical) position and stabilised. This is best achieved with a rigid collar of appropriate size supplemented, for example, with sandbags on each side of the head and with forehead tape. If gross spinal deformity is left uncorrected and splinted, the cervical cord may sustain further injury from unrelieved compression. Thoracolumbar injury must also be assumed and treated by carefully straightening the trunk and correcting rotation. During turning or lifting, it is vital that the whole spine is maintained in the neutral position. While positioning the patient, relevant information can be obtained from witnesses and a brief assessment of superficial wounds may suggest the mechanism of injury—for example, wounds of the forehead often accompany hyperextension injuries of the cervical spine.

Although the spine is best immobilised by placing the patient supine, and this position is important for resuscitation and the rapid assessment of life threatening injuries, unconscious patients on their backs are at risk of passive gastric regurgitation and aspiration of vomit. This can be avoided by endotracheal intubation, which is the ideal method of securing the airway in an unconscious casualty. If intubation cannot be performed the patient should be "log rolled" carefully into a modified lateral position 70-80° from prone with the head supported in the neutral position by the underlying arm. This posture allows secretions to drain freely from the mouth, and a rigid collar helps to minimise neck movement. Log rolling should be performed by four people in a coordinated manner ensuring that unnecessary movement does not occur in any part of the spine. The prone position is unsatisfactory as it may severely embarrass respiration, particularly in the tetraplegic patient. The semiprone recovery position is also contraindicated, as it results in rotation of the neck.

Patency of the airway and adequate oxygenation must take priority in unconscious patients. The mouth should be opened by chin lift or jaw thrust, cleared of debris, an oropharyngeal airway inserted, and oxygen given. With care, endotracheal intubation is usually safe in patients with injuries to the spinal cord. Intubation may be performed at the scene of the accident or later in the hospital receiving room, depending on the patient's level of consciousness and the ability of the attending doctor or paramedic. Orotracheal intubation is rendered more safe if an assistant holds the head and minimises neck movement. Blind intubation (orotracheal or nasotracheal) may be undertaken by experienced doctors if it can be accomplished without rotating the neck, but this requires expertise.

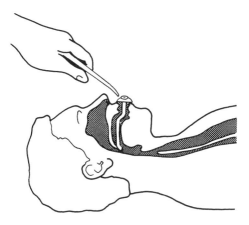

Suction: beware of vagal reflex stimulation.

Clinical features of spinal cord injury

- Pain in the neck or back, often radiating because of nerve root irritation

- Sensory disturbance distal to neurological level

- Weakness or flaccid paralysis below this level

Narcotic analgesics should be avoided if possible in patients with cervical and upper thoracic injuries

If possible, suction should be avoided in tetraplegic patients as it may stimulate the vagal reflex, aggravate pre-existing bradycardia, and occasionally precipitate cardiac arrest (to be discussed later). The risk of unwanted vagal effects can be minimised if atropine is administered beforehand in addition to oxygen. In hospital, flexible fibreoptic instruments may provide the ideal solution to the intubation of patients with unstable cervical injury.

Once the airway is protected intravenous access should be established in case cardiopulmonary support is required, but clinicians should remember that in uncomplicated cases of high spinal cord injury patients may be hypotensive due to sympathetic paralysis and may easily be overinfused. If respiration and circulation are satisfactory patients can be examined briefly where they lie. A basic examination should include measurement of pulse and blood pressure, brief assessment of level of consciousness and pupillary responses, examination of chest and abdomen for signs of gross trauma, and passive limb movement to detect fracture or dislocation. Spinal cord injury may be suggested by spinal deformity, increased interspinous gap, diaphragmatic breathing due to intercostal paralysis (seen in patients with tetraplegia or high thoracic paraplegia), and flaccidity with areflexia in the paralysed limbs.

The conscious patient

The diagnosis of spinal cord injury rests on the symptoms and signs of pain in the spine, sensory disturbance, and weakness or flaccid paralysis. In conscious patients with these features resuscitative measures should again be given priority. At the same time a brief history can be obtained, which will help to localise the level of spinal trauma and identify other injuries that may further compromise the nutrition of the damaged spinal cord by producing hypoxia or hypovolaemic shock. A short general examination should be undertaken and a basic neurological assessment made by asking patients to what extent they can feel or move their limbs.

Analgesia

In patients with low spinal cord injuries opioid analgesics are usually safe, but in cervical and upper thoracic injuries where ventilation is already impaired, they should be avoided in the first instance if possible, particularly as chest and head injuries often coexist. If pain is uncontrollable without their use, small, intravenous doses of opioid analgesics are recommended, the dose being kept to a minimum to control symptoms without causing respiratory depression. Mild analgesics and intramuscular non-steroidal anti-inflammatory drugs are often effective and relatively safe, but buprenorphine is best avoided because its effects will be only partially reversed by naloxone if respiratory depression develops.

EVACUATION AND INITIAL MANAGEMENT AT HOSPITAL

Andrew Swain, David Grundy

Evacuation and transfer to hospital

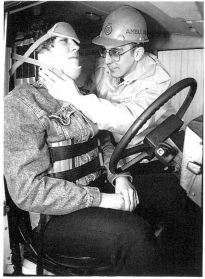

Patient being removed from a vehicle with a semirigid collar and spinal immobiliser (Kendrick extrication device) in position.

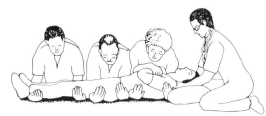

A coordinated spinal lift.

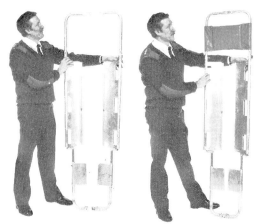

Scoop stretcher.

If casualties are trapped in a vehicle it may be safer to apply a spinal board or immobiliser before moving them. These devices should be used in conjunction with a semirigid collar of appropriate size to prevent movement of any part of the spine. If the correct collars or splints are not available it may be necessary to improvise, but in such circumstances manual immobilisation of the head is the safest option.

The patient should be moved by four people: one responsible for the head and neck, one for the shoulders and chest, one for the hips and abdomen, and one for the legs. The person holding the head and neck directs movement.

The patient should be placed supine on a firm stretcher if conscious or intubated. A "scoop" stretcher is ideal as it can be slotted together around the casualty with minimum disturbance. To stabilise the neck a semirigid collar must be applied with sandbags on each side of the head and with forehead tape to prevent rotation. The only exception to this is the physically uncooperative or thrashing patient, who may manipulate the cervical spine from below if the head and neck are fixed in position. Such a patient should be fitted with only a semirigid collar and restrained as much as possible. If the airway is unprotected, the modified lateral position is recommended with the head supported and neutral. In the absence of life threatening injury patients should be transported slowly by ambulance, for reasons of comfort as well as to avoid further trauma to the spinal cord. They should be taken to the nearest major accident and emergency department but must be repeatedly assessed en route; in particular, vital functions must be monitored. In transit, patients should not be left unattended, and the head and neck must be maintained in the neutral position at all times. If unintubated supine patients start to vomit, it is safer to tip them head down and apply oropharyngeal suction than to attempt an uncoordinated turn into the lateral position.

Hard objects should be removed from patients' pockets, and anaesthetic areas should be protected to prevent pressure sores developing.

The usual vasomotor responses to changes of temperature are impaired in tetraplegia and high paraplegia because the sympathetic system is paralysed. The patient is therefore poikilothermic, and hypothermia is a particular risk when these patients are transported during the winter months. Blankets and thermal reflector sheets are often needed to maintain body temperature.

When the injury has been sustained in an inaccessible location or the patient has to be evacuated over a long distance, transfer by helicopter has been shown to reduce mortality and morbidity. If a helicopter is used, the possibility of immediate transfer to the regional spinal injuries unit should be considered, after discussion with that unit.

Initial management at the receiving hospital

<table>
<tr><td>

Associated injuries

Spinal cord injury is accompanied by:

Head injuries (coma of more than 6 hours' duration; or skull fracture present) in 7%

Chest injuries (requiring active treatment; or rib fractures) in 20%

Abdominal injuries (requiring laparotomy) in 2·5%

Multiple injuries (including skeletal, other than the above categories) in 24%

Figures derived from new injury admissions to Duke of Cornwall Spinal Treatment Centre 1989-91

</td></tr>
</table>

When the patient arrives at the nearest major accident unit a detailed history must be obtained and a full general and neurological examination performed. The general examination must be thorough because spinal trauma is often associated with multiple injuries, commonly affecting the head and chest. Specific signs of spinal injury should be sought, including local bruising and tenderness, deformity of the spine—for example, a gibbus or an increased interspinous gap—and priapism, which invariably indicates a high spinal cord lesion. The patient must be subjected to a coordinated log roll for proper and safe assessment of the back.

Diagnosis of intra-abdominal injury may be very difficult in patients with high cord lesions (above the seventh thoracic segment) during the initial phase of spinal shock, when paralytic ileus and abdominal distension are usual. Abdominal sensation is impaired, and this, together with the flaccid paralysis, means that the classic signs of an intra-abdominal emergency may be absent. The signs of peritoneal irritation do not develop and, in these circumstances, peritoneal lavage is recommended.

The neurological examination must include assessment of the following:

(a) sensation to pin prick (spinothalamic tracts);

(b) sensation to fine touch and joint position sense (posterior columns);

(c) power of muscle groups according to the Medical Research Council scale (corticospinal tracts);

(d) reflexes (including abdominal, anal, and bulbocavernosus reflexes);

(e) cranial nerve function.

By examining the dermatomes and myotomes in this way, the level and completeness of neurological damage are assessed. The last segment of normal spinal cord function, as judged by clinical examination, is referred to as the neurological level of the lesion. This often, but not necessarily, corresponds with the level of bony injury. Sensory or motor sparing may be present below this level—an incomplete lesion.

The neurological and bony diagnoses should both be recorded—for example, "incomplete paraplegia below T8 (or T8I) due to a fracture of T7" or "complete tetraplegia below C6 (or C6C) due to a fracture of C6."

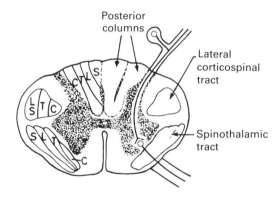

Posterior columns

Lateral corticospinal tract

Spinothalamic tract

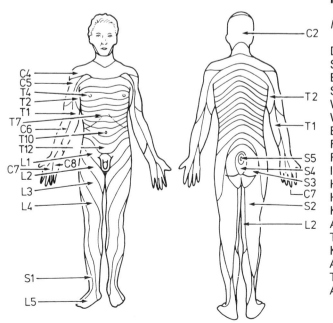

Myotomes	Reflexes	
Muscle group	*nerve supply*	
Diaphragm	C(3),4,(5)	
Shoulder abductors	C5	
Elbow flexors	C5,6	Biceps jerk C5,6
Supinators/pronators	C6	Supinator jerk C6
Wrist extensors	C6	
Wrist flexors	C7	
Elbow extensors	C7	Triceps jerk C7
Finger extensors	C7	
Finger flexors	C8	
Intrinsic hand muscles	T1	Abdominal reflex T8-12
Hip flexors	L1,2	
Hip adductors	L2,3	
Knee extensors	L3,4	Knee jerk L3,4
Ankle dorsiflexors	L4,5	
Toe extensors	L5	
Knee flexors	L4,5 S1	
Ankle plantar flexors	S1,2	Ankle jerk S1,2
Toe flexors	S1,2	
Anal sphincter	S2,3,4	Bulbocavernosus reflex S3,4
		Anal reflex S5
		Plantar reflex

Spinal shock

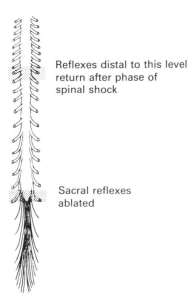

Reflexes distal to this level return after phase of spinal shock

Sacral reflexes ablated

After severe spinal cord injury, spinal shock with generalised flaccidity below the level of the lesion supervenes and, although reflex activity may initially be present, even this disappears after a period. Spinal shock may last from a few hours to several weeks. Its end is marked by a return of reflex activity in the spinal cord, when the lesion is above the sacral segments—that is, when there is an upper motor neurone lesion. The anal and bulbocavernosus reflexes are usually the first to return. In lower motor neurone lesions affecting either the conus medullaris or cauda equina, reflexes remain absent unless neurological recovery occurs.

The anal and bulbocavernosus reflexes both depend on intact sacral reflex arcs. The anal reflex is an externally visible contraction of the anal sphincter in response to perianal pin prick. The bulbocavernosus reflex is a similar contraction of the anal sphincter felt with the examining finger in response to squeezing the glans penis. If the sacral segments are spared in an incomplete injury these reflexes may persist throughout the phase of spinal shock, and the likelihood of a return of bladder and bowel control is increased. However, the bulbocavernosus reflex and also the plantar response are not always reliable indicators in the diagnosis and prognosis of acute spinal cord injury.

Incomplete spinal cord injury

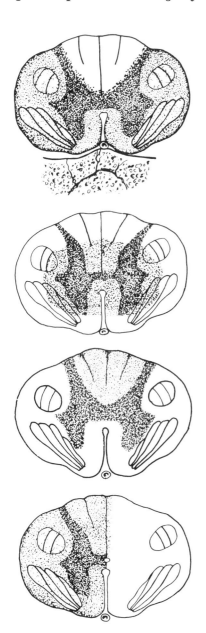

Assessment of the level and completeness of the spinal cord injury allows a prognosis to be made. If the lesion is complete from the outset—that is, if there is no sign of spinal cord function below the level of injury—recovery is far less likely than in an incomplete lesion. There are recognised patterns of incomplete cord injury, and variations of these may present in the accident and emergency department.

Anterior cord syndrome—The anterior part of the spinal cord is usually injured by a flexion-rotation force to the spine producing an anterior dislocation or by a compression fracture of the vertebral body with bony encroachment on the vertebral canal. There is often anterior spinal artery compression so that the corticospinal and spinothalamic tracts are damaged by a combination of direct trauma and ischaemia. This results in loss of power as well as reduced pain and temperature sensation below the lesion.

Central cord syndrome—This is typically seen in older patients with cervical spondylosis. A hyperextension injury, often from relatively minor trauma, compresses the spinal cord between the irregular osteophytic vertebral body and the intervertebral disc anteriorly and the thickened ligamentum flavum posteriorly. The more centrally situated cervical tracts supplying the arms suffer the brunt of the injury so that classically there is a flaccid (lower motor neurone) weakness of the arms and relatively strong but spastic (upper motor neurone) leg function. Sacral sensation and bladder and bowel function are often partially spared.

Posterior cord syndrome—This syndrome is most commonly seen in hyperextension injuries with fractures of the posterior elements of the vertebrae. There is contusion of the posterior columns so the patient may have good power and pain and temperature sensation but there is sometimes profound ataxia due to the loss of proprioception, which can make walking very difficult.

Brown-Séquard syndrome—Classically resulting from stab injuries but also common in lateral mass fractures of the vertebrae, the signs of the Brown-Séquard syndrome are those of a hemisection of the spinal cord. Power is reduced or absent but pain and temperature sensation are relatively normal on the side of the injury because the spinothalamic tract crosses over to the opposite side of the cord. The uninjured side therefore has good power but reduced or absent sensation to pin prick and temperature.

The final phase in the diagnosis of spinal trauma entails radiology of the spine to assess the level and nature of the injury.

RADIOLOGICAL INVESTIGATIONS

David Grundy, Andrew Swain

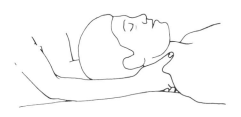

Radiological investigation of a high standard is crucial to the correct diagnosis of a spinal injury. Sandbags and collars are not always radiolucent, and clearer radiographs may be obtained if these are removed after preliminary films (normally a chest radiograph and a lateral view of the cervical spine) have been taken. Most accident departments rely on the use of mobile radiographic equipment for investigating seriously ill patients, but the quality of films obtained in this way is invariably inferior. If the patient's condition is otherwise satisfactory, but a spinal injury is suspected, radiographs should be taken in the radiology department with a doctor in attendance to ensure that spinal movement is minimised.

Cervical injuries

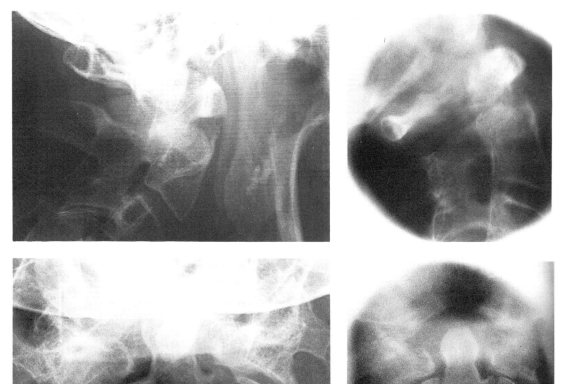

Fracture of odontoid process. The diagnosis is not obvious from the standard views (left) because of poor definition, but a clue is the obvious posterior displacement of the anterior arch of the atlas on the lateral radiograph. Tomography (right) shows the fracture clearly.

The first and most important radiograph to be taken of a patient with a suspected cervical cord injury is the lateral view. This is more likely than the anteroposterior view to show spinal damage and can be taken in the accident department without moving supine patients. Other views are best obtained in the radiology department. Anteroposterior radiographs must be taken, including an open mouth view of the odontoid process.

Radiological investigations

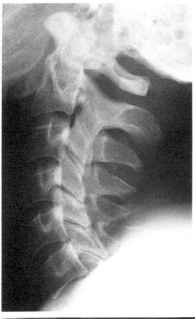 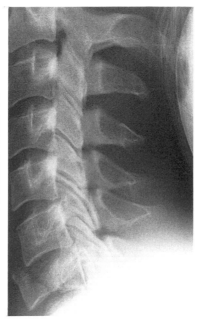

The lateral view should be repeated if the original radiograph does not show the whole of the cervical spine. Failure to insist on this often results in injuries of the lower cervical spine being missed. The lower cervical vertebrae are often obscured by the shoulders unless these are depressed by traction on both arms. The traction must be stopped if it produces pain in the neck. If the lower cervical spine is still not seen, a supine "swimmer's" view with the central ray directed at right angles to the longitudinal axis of the vertebral column (usually angled 10-15° cranially) should be taken. With the near shoulder depressed and the arm next to the cassette abducted, abnormalities as far down as the first or second thoracic vertebra will usually be shown. Occasionally lateral tomography is necessary to show the cervicothoracic junction.

Compression fracture of C7, missed initially because of failure to show the entire cervical spine.

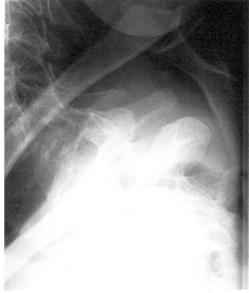 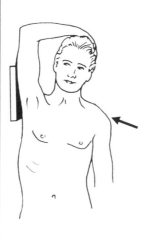

Left: swimmer's view—the patient is supine. Far left: swimmer's view—note the dislocation of C6-7, seen immediately below the clavicular shadow.

In the cervical spine dislocation and fractures may both be seen on the lateral radiograph. Anterior vertebral displacement of less than half the diameter of the vertebral body suggests unilateral facet dislocation; displacement greater than this indicates a bilateral facet dislocation. Displacement of a spinous process from the midline on the anteroposterior film is explained by vertebral rotation secondary to unilateral facet dislocation, the spinous process being displaced towards the side of the dislocation. In bilateral facet dislocation the spinous processes are in line. With a unilateral facet dislocation the spine is relatively stable, especially if maintained in extension. With a bilateral facet dislocation the spine is always unstable, and the patient therefore requires extreme care when being handled.

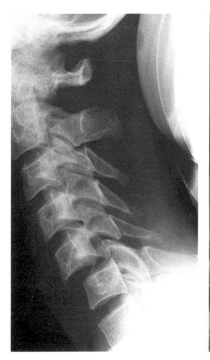 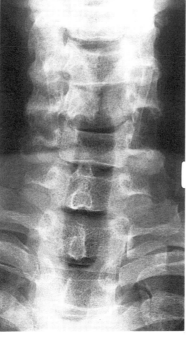

Lateral and anteroposterior films in C5-6 unilateral facet dislocation. Note the less than half vertebral body slip in the lateral view, and the lack of alignment of spinous processes, owing to rotation, in the anteroposterior view.

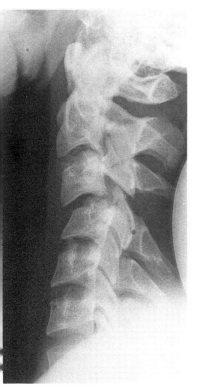
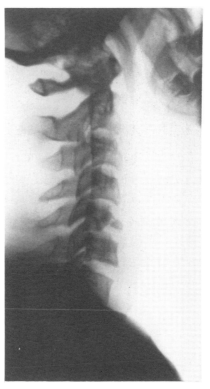

Other useful radiological signs should be sought when bony abnormalities are minimal or absent. Thus on the lateral radiograph the soft tissue shadow of a prevertebral haematoma may be evident, and a widened gap between adjacent spinous processes denotes rupture of the posterior cervical ligamentous complex. This is an unstable injury, often associated with vertebral subluxation and crush fracture of the vertebral body. Atlantoaxial subluxation may be identified by an increased gap (more than 2·5 mm in adults and 4 mm in children) between the odontoid process and the anterior arch of the atlas on the lateral radiograph.

Left: C3-4 dislocation, postreduction film showing continuing instability because of posterior ligamentous damage. Right: Teardrop fracture of C5 with retropulsion of vertebral body into spinal canal.

Fractures of the anteroinferior margin of the vertebral body ("teardrop" fractures) are often associated with an unstable flexion injury and sometimes retropulsion of the vertebral body or disc material into the spinal canal. Similarly, flakes of bone may be avulsed from the anterosuperior margin of the vertebral body by the anterior longitudinal ligament in severe extension injuries.

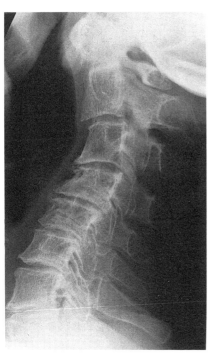
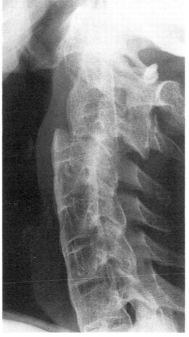

In older patients with cervical spondylosis and tetraplegia resulting from a hyperextension injury, there is often no fracture or dislocation to be seen. Likewise in children, because their spines are more mobile, traction injury to the spinal cord may occur without evidence of bony damage. Pathological changes in the spine—for example, ankylosing spondylitis or rheumatoid arthritis—may predispose to bony damage after relatively minor trauma.

Left: central cord syndrome without bony damage, in a patient with cervical spondylosis. Right: transverse fracture through C3 in a patient with ankylosing spondylitis.

Radiological investigations

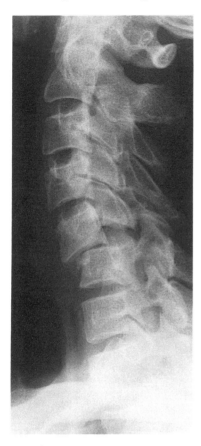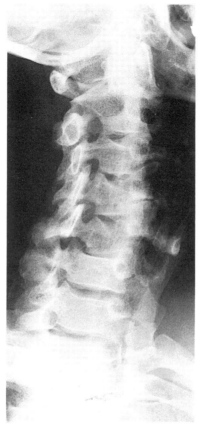

Oblique radiographs are not routinely obtained, but they do help to confirm the presence of subluxation or dislocation and indicate whether the right or left facets (apophyseal joints), or both, are affected.

The 45° supine oblique view shows the intervertebral foramina and the facets, but a better view for the facets is one taken with the patient log rolled 22·5° from the horizontal.

Flexion and extension views of the cervical spine may be taken if the patient has no neurological symptoms or signs and initial radiographs are normal but an unstable (ligamentous) injury is nevertheless suspected. To obtain these radiographs, flexion and extension of the whole neck must be performed by the patient under the supervision of an experienced doctor. Movement must cease if neurological symptoms are precipitated.

The 22½° oblique view of the right facet joints (left) shows clearly the facet dislocation at the C5-6 level, less obvious in the 45° oblique view (right), which however shows a malalignment of the intervertebral foramina.

Thoracolumbar injuries

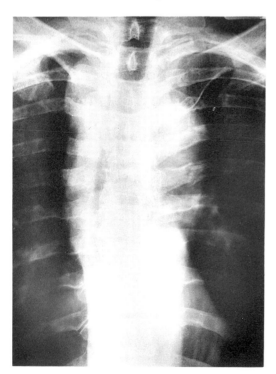

Severe trauma is required to damage the thoracic, lumbar, and sacral segments of the spinal cord, and the skeletal injury is usually evident on the standard anteroposterior and horizontal beam lateral radiographs. Signs of instability, particularly fracture through the posterior facet joints or pedicles, are more easily seen on the lateral radiograph. Showing detail in the thoracic spine can be extremely difficult, however, particularly in the upper four vertebrae, and lateral tomography is sometimes required for better definition. Instability in thoracic spinal injuries may also be caused by sternal or bilateral rib fractures, as the anterior splinting effect of these structures will be lost.

A haematoma in the posterior mediastinum is often seen around the fracture site, particularly in the anteroposterior view, and if there is any suspicion that these appearances might be due to traumatic aortic dissection an arch aortogram will be required.

Patient with fracture of T5 with widening of mediastinum due to a prevertebral haematoma, initially diagnosed as traumatic dissection of the aorta, for which he underwent aortography.

Other investigations

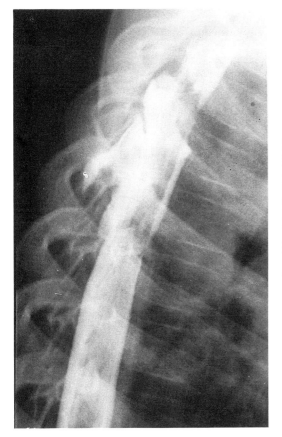

Emergency myelography after spinal cord injury is of limited value, particularly as the procedure may require the patient to be turned in different positions, with risk of further trauma to the spinal cord. Myelography has been used to try to identify causes of cord compression, particularly in patients with progressive neurological deficit, or those with no radiological evidence of trauma. Interpretation is difficult, however, and because a computed tomogram (CT scan) can show traumatic disc prolapse and loose bony fragments within the spinal canal, myelography is rarely indicated. With the advent of magnetic resonance imaging (MRI), spinal cord compression and damage can be shown much more clearly.

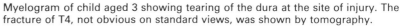

Myelogram of child aged 3 showing tearing of the dura at the site of injury. The fracture of T4, not obvious on standard views, was shown by tomography.

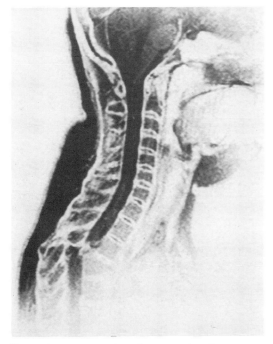

Magnetic resonance imaging scan showing transection of the spinal cord associated with a fracture of T4.

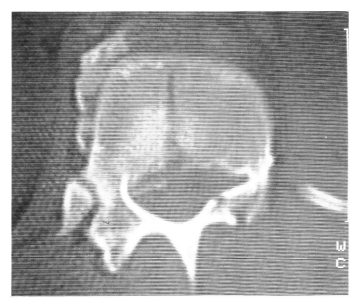

Computed tomogram of T12 showing a compression fracture of the vertebral body with displacement of bony fragments into the spinal canal and damage in the region of the posterior facet joints.

EARLY MANAGEMENT AND COMPLICATIONS—I

David Grundy, Andrew Swain

Respiratory complications

Respiratory insufficiency is common in patients with injuries of the cervical cord. If the neurological lesion is complete the patient will have paralysed intercostal muscles and will have to rely on diaphragmatic respiration. Partial paralysis of the diaphragm may also be present, either from the outset or after 24-48 hours if ascending post-traumatic cord oedema develops. In patients with injuries of the thoracic spine, respiratory impairment often results from associated rib fractures, haemopneumothorax, or pulmonary contusion; there may also be a varying degree of intercostal paralysis depending on the neurological level of the lesion.

Sputum retention occurs readily during the first few days after injury, particularly in patients with high lesions and in those with associated chest injury. The inability to produce an effective cough impairs the clearing of secretions and commonly leads to atelectasis. Cardiac arrest after spinal cord injury is often secondary to respiratory failure. Abnormal distribution of gases and blood (ventilation-perfusion mismatch) also occurs in the lungs of tetraplegic patients, producing further respiratory impairment.

Regular chest physiotherapy with assisted coughing and breathing exercises is vital to prevent atelectasis and pulmonary infection. Respiratory function should be monitored by measuring the vital capacity and arterial blood gases. A vital capacity of less than 1 litre should alert clinicians, and a fall to 500-600 ml may necessitate endotracheal intubation and ventilation. Once this step has been taken the inspired air must be humified; otherwise secretions will become viscid and difficult to clear. If atelectasis necessitates bronchoscopy this is a safe procedure performed with modern fibreoptic instruments, which can be used without undue movement of the patient's neck. If the patient is already intubated the fibreoptic bronchoscope can be passed down the endotracheal tube. Tracheostomy is best avoided in the first instance, as ventilation is sometimes needed for a few days only. Minitracheostomy is useful if the problem is purely one of retained secretions.

A patient whose respiratory function is initially satisfactory after injury but then deteriorates should regain satisfactory ventilatory capacity once spinal cord oedema subsides. Artificial ventilation should therefore not be withheld, except perhaps in the elderly and infirm. If there is a risk of deterioration in respiratory function during transit, an anaesthetist must accompany the patient.

With increasing public awareness of cardiopulmonary resuscitation and the routine attendance of paramedics at accidents, patients with high cervical injuries and complete phrenic nerve paralysis are surviving. They often require long term ventilatory support, and this can be achieved either mechanically or electronically by phrenic nerve pacing. The necessity for ventilation should be no bar to the patient returning home, and patients are now surviving with a satisfactory quality of life on domiciliary ventilation.

Causes of respiratory insufficiency

In tetraplegia:

Intercostal paralysis

Partial phrenic nerve palsy—immediate

　　　　　　　　　　　　　—delayed

Impaired ability to expectorate

Ventilation-perfusion mismatch

In paraplegia:

Variable intercostal paralysis according to
　　level of injury

Associated chest injuries

　　　　　　　—rib fractures

　　　　　　　—pulmonary contusion

　　　　　　　—haemopneumothorax

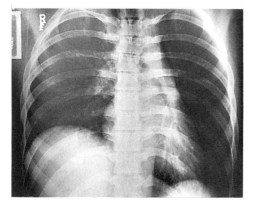

Right diaphragmatic paralysis resulting from ascending cord oedema developing 48 hours after the patient had sustained complete tetraplegia below C4, because of C3-4 dislocation.

Cardiovascular complications

> **Beware of overinfusion in patients with neurogenic shock**

> **Treat**
> Bradycardia <50 beats/min
> Hypotension <80 mm Hg systolic or adequate urinary excretion not maintained

Haemorrhage from associated injuries is the commonest cause of post-traumatic shock and must be treated. However, it must be realised that in traumatic tetraplegia the thoracolumbar (T1-L2) sympathetic outflow is interrupted. Vagal tone is therefore unopposed and the patient becomes hypotensive and bradycardic. Even in paraplegia sympathetic paralysis below the lesion can produce hypotension—neurogenic shock. If shock is purely neurogenic in origin, patients can mistakenly be given large volumes of intravenous fluid. Pulmonary oedema resulting from overinfusion was the commonest cause of death in patients with spinal cord injury in the Vietnam war.

Pharyngeal suction and endotracheal intubation stimulate the vagus, producing bradycardia, which may result in cardiac arrest. To prevent this it is wise to give atropine or glycopyrronium in addition to oxygen before suction and intubation are undertaken and also whenever the heart rate falls below 50 beats/minute. Clinicians, however, must be aware of the possible toxic effects when the standard dose of 0·6 mg atropine is used repeatedly. If the systolic blood pressure cannot maintain adequate perfusion pressure to produce an acceptable flow of urine after any hypovolaemia has been corrected then inotropic medication with dopamine should be started.

Cardiac arrest due to sudden hyperkalaemia after the use of a depolarising agent such as suxamethonium for endotracheal intubation is a risk in patients with spinal cord injury, and this drug should not be given from three days to nine months after injury. If muscle relaxation is required for intubation during this period a non-depolarising muscle relaxant such as pancuronium is indicated to avoid the risk of hyperkalaemic cardiac arrest.

The anatomy of spinal cord injury

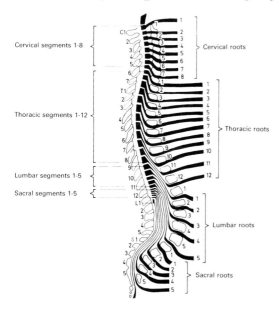

The radiographic appearances of the spine after injury are not a reliable guide to the severity of spinal cord damage. They represent the final or "recoil" position of the vertebrae and do not necessarily indicate the forces generated in the injury. The spinal cord ends at the lower border of the first lumbar vertebra in adults, the remainder of the spinal canal being occupied by the nerve roots of the cauda equina. There is greater room for the neural structures in the cervical and lumbar canals, but in the thoracic region the spinal cord diameter and that of the neural canal more nearly approximate. The blood supply of the cervical spinal cord is good, whereas that of the thoracic cord, especially at its midpoint, is relatively poor. These factors may explain the greater preponderance of complete lesions seen after injuries to the thoracic spine. The initial injury is mechanical, but there is usually an early ischaemic lesion that may rapidly progress to cord necrosis. Extension of this, often many segments below the level of the lesion, accounts for the observation that on occasion patients have lower motor neurone or flaccid paralysis when upper neurone or spastic paralysis would have been expected from the site of the bony injury. Because of the potential for regeneration of peripheral nerves, neurological recovery is unpredictable in lesions of the cauda equina.

The spinal injury: cervical spine

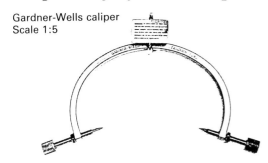

Gardner-Wells caliper
Scale 1:5

Patients with injuries of the cervical spine should initially be managed by skeletal traction. Applied through skull calipers, traction is aimed at reducing any fracture or dislocation, relieving pressure on the cord in the case of burst fractures, and splinting the spine.

Of the various skull calipers available, the Gardner-Wells is the most suitable for inserting in the accident and emergency department. Local anaesthetic is infiltrated into the scalp about 2·5 cms above the pinna, at the site of the maximum bitemporal diameter, and the caliper is then screwed into the scalp to grip the outer table of the skull. No incisions need be made, and spring loading of one of the

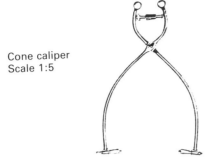

Cone caliper
Scale 1:5

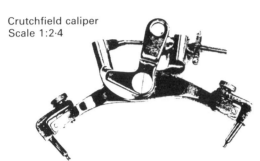

Crutchfield caliper
Scale 1:2·4

screws determines when the correct tension has been reached. The University of Virginia caliper is similar in action and easily applied. The Cone caliper is satisfactory but requires small scalp incisions and the drilling of 1 mm impressions in the outer table of the skull. Insertion too far anteriorly interferes with temporalis function and causes trismus. The Crutchfield caliper is inserted into the outer table of the vault of the skull through incisions 5 cm from the midline and in the plane of the external auditory meati. Although its small size and site of insertion may facilitate turning of the patient, it is not recommended because of the high incidence of complications. Unless correctly inserted it tends to fall out, and the securing pins may penetrate the inner table of the skull.

When the upper cervical spine is injured less traction is required for reduction and stabilisation. Usually 1 to 2 kg is enough for stabilisation; if more weight is used overdistraction at the site of injury may cause neurological deterioration. Specific injuries of the upper cervical spine and the cervicothoracic junction will be discussed later.

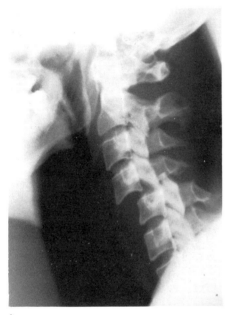

1

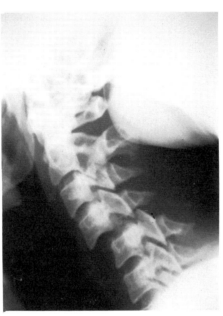

2

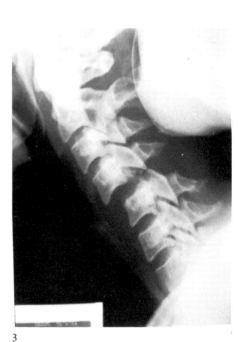

3

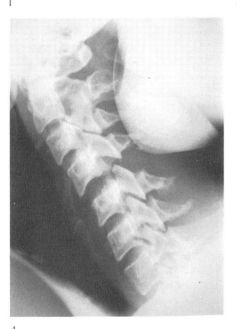

4

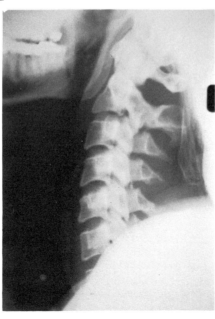

5

Illustrations 1 to 5 show reduction of a C4-5 bilateral facet dislocation due to severe flexion injury. Increasing traction weight was applied with the neck in flexion for $3\frac{1}{2}$ hours to 25 kg (illustrations 1 to 4). Illustration 5 shows the final position after 4 hours with head extended and weight reduced to 4 kg traction. Improvement in neurological level from C5 to C6.

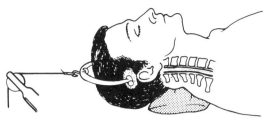

Skull traction using Gardner-Wells caliper, with neck roll in position.

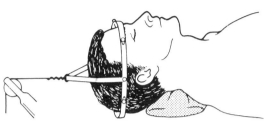

Halo applied with the bale arm—an alternative approach to skull traction if early mobilisation into a halo brace is being considered.

A traction force of 3 to 5 kg is normally applied to the calipers in fractures of the lower cervical spine without dislocation. A neck roll (not a sandbag) should be placed behind the neck to maintain the normal cervical lordosis. Pressure sores of the scalp in the occipital region are common, and care must be taken to cushion the occiput when positioning the patient. When necessary a suitably covered fluid filled plastic bag can be used, having ensured that there is no matted hair that could act as a source of pressure. If the spine is dislocated reduction can usually be achieved by increasing the weight by about 4 kg every 30 minutes (sometimes up to a total of 25 kg) with the neck in flexion until the facets are disengaged. The neck is then extended and the traction decreased to maintenance weight. The patient must be examined neurologically before each increment, and the traction force must be reduced immediately if the neurology deteriorates.

Manipulation under general anaesthesia is an alternative method of reduction, but, although complete neurological recovery has been reported after this procedure, there have been adverse effects in some patients and manipulation should only be attempted by people with experience. Such reductions may be helped by the use of an image intensifier.

Halo traction is a useful alternative to skull calipers, particularly in patients with incomplete tetraplegia, and conversion to a halo brace permits early mobilisation.

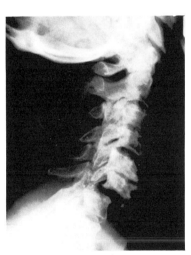
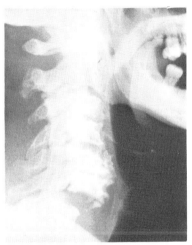

Left: bilateral facet dislocation in a patient with associated cervical spondylosis. Right: incorrect traction—too great a weight and head in extension—leading to distraction with neurological deterioration.

Skull traction is a satisfactory treatment for unstable injuries of the cervical spine in the early stages, but when the spinal cord lesion is incomplete early operative fusion may be indicated to prevent further neurological damage. The decision to operate may sometimes be made before the patient is transferred to the spinal injuries unit, but if so the spinal unit should be consulted and management planned jointly.

Another indication for operation is an open wound, such as that following a gunshot or stab injury, exploration or debridement of which should be performed.

Skull traction is unnecessary for patients with cervical spondylosis who sustain a hyperextension injury with tetraplegia but have no fracture or dislocation. In these circumstances the patient should be nursed with the head in slight flexion but otherwise free from restriction.

Thoracolumbar spine

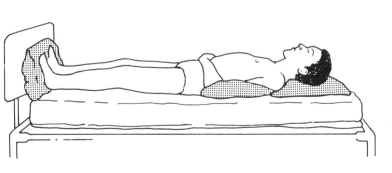

Most thoracolumbar injuries are due to flexion-rotation forces. The standard treatment for thoracolumbar injuries associated with cord damage is conservative, with the patient supported to maintain the correct posture. In practice a pillow under the lumbar spine to preserve normal lordosis is usually all that is necessary. Dislocations of the thoracic and lumbar spine are often reduced by this technique of "postural reduction".

However, internal fixation is recommended in some patients with unstable fracture dislocations to prevent further cord or nerve root damage, correct deformity, and facilitate nursing, but as yet there is no convincing evidence that internal fixation aids neurological recovery.

The illustration of the relation between spinal cord segments and vertebral bodies is reproduced by permission from Haymaker W. *Bing's Local Diagnosis in Neurological Disease*. C V Mosby.

EARLY MANAGEMENT AND COMPLICATIONS—II

David Grundy, Andrew Swain

The urinary tract

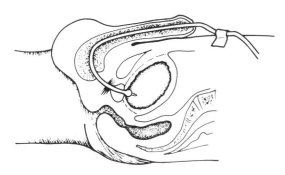

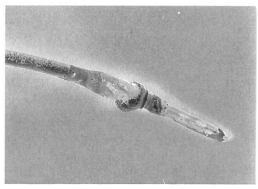

Encrustation of a suprapubic catheter.

After a severe spinal cord injury the bladder is initially acontractile. The volume of urine in the bladder should never be allowed to exceed 500 ml because overstretching the detrusor muscle can delay the return of bladder function. If the patient is transferred to a spinal injuries unit within a few hours after injury it may be possible to defer catheterisation until then, but if the patient drank a large volume of fluid before injury this is unwise. In these circumstances, and in patients with multiple injuries, the safest course is to pass a small bore (12-14 Ch) 5–10 ml balloon latex, or preferably silicone, Foley catheter. In men this should be strapped to the anterior abdominal wall in the midline to produce a gentle curve of the urethra and thus minimise pressure on the posterior urethral wall, reducing the risk of periurethral abscess and fistula formation. In women the catheter is secured to the thigh.

A latex catheter must be changed weekly, though a silicone catheter may be left in situ for up to six weeks. A bladder washout with Suby-G solution (containing citric acid 3·23%) twice a week is helpful in preventing stone encrustation on the balloon of the catheter. Encrustation is particularly likely to occur in the weeks after spinal cord injury because of hypercalciuria secondary to paralysis and immobility, but the small (5–10 ml) balloon minimises this risk. If encrustation forms on the balloon then fragments tend to break off, producing "eggshell" calculi in the bladder, which may block the catheter and also predispose to urinary tract infection. With hypercalciuria, bladder calculi may also occur even if an indwelling catheter is not being used. On admission to the spinal injuries unit intermittent urethral catheterisation or fine bore suprapubic catheterisation can be started.

With intermittent catheterisation the patient is normally catheterised every six hours, with a 12-14 Ch Nelaton catheter, using a rigorously sterile technique. To prevent overdistension of the bladder, fluids initially need to be restricted so as to produce a urinary output of not more than 1500 ml in 24 hours, until the patient starts voiding spontaneously. At this stage the fluid intake can be increased. The great advantage of the suprapubic catheter is that fluid restriction is unnecessary; indeed, a high fluid intake should be maintained in an effort to reduce the incidence of infection and stone formation, although the risk of encrustation still remains.

The gastrointestinal tract

> **Beware of paralytic ileus: patients should receive intravenous fluids for at least the first 48 hours after injury**

The patient should receive intravenous fluids for at least the first 48 hours, as paralytic ileus usually accompanies a severe spinal injury. A nasogastric tube is passed and oral fluids are forbidden until normal bowel sounds return. If paralytic ileus becomes prolonged the abdominal distension splints the diaphragm and, particularly in tetraplegic patients, this may precipitate a respiratory crisis if not relieved by nasogastric aspiration. If a tetraplegic patient vomits, gastric contents are easily aspirated because the patient cannot cough effectively. Ileus may also be precipitated by an excessive lumbar lordosis if too bulky a lumbar pillow is used for thoracolumbar injuries.

Acute peptic ulceration, with haemorrhage or perforation, is an uncommon but dangerous complication after spinal cord injury, and for this reason giving ranitidine should be started as soon as possible after injury and continued for at least three weeks. When perforation occurs it often presents a week after injury with referred pain to the shoulder, but during the stage of spinal shock guarding and rigidity will be absent and tachycardia may not develop. A lateral decubitus abdominal film usually shows free gas in the peritoneal cavity.

The skin and pressure areas

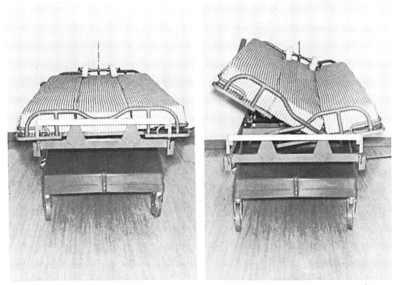

Egerton turning and tilting bed to show mechanism for (left) supine position and (right) left lateral position.

When the patient is transferred from trolley to bed the whole of the back must be inspected for bruising, abrasions, or signs of pressure on the skin. The patient should be turned every two hours between supine and right and left lateral positions to prevent pressure sores, and the skin should be inspected at each turn. Manual turning can be achieved on a standard hospital bed, by lifting patients to one side, using the method described in the chapter on nursing, and then log rolling them into the lateral position. Alternatively, the electrically driven Egerton turning and tilting bed can be used. Another convenient solution is the Stryker frame, in which a patient is "sandwiched" between anterior and posterior sections, which can then be turned between the supine and prone positions by the inbuilt circular turning mechanism, but tetraplegic patients may not tolerate the prone position.

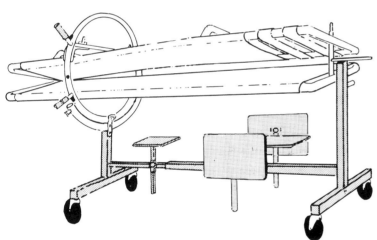

Stryker frame.

> **Pillows:**
> Protect against pressure sores
> Support the site of injury
> Maintain spinal contour
> Help prevent contractures

Nursing care requires the use of pillows to separate the legs, maintain alignment of the spine, and prevent the formation of contractures. In injuries of the cervical spine a neck roll is used to maintain cervical lordosis. A lumbar pillow maintains lumbar lordosis in thoracolumbar injuries. Foot drop and equinous contracture are prevented by placing a vertical pillow between the foot of the bed and the soles of the feet.

Prophylaxis against thromboembolism

Newly injured tetraplegic or paraplegic patients have a high risk of developing thromboembolic complications. The incidence of pulmonary embolism reaches a maximum in the third week after injury and is the commonest cause of death in patients who survive the period immediately after the injury.

If there are no other injuries or medical contraindications, anticoagulation should be started 24-36 hours after the accident. Prophylaxis against deep vein thrombosis and pulmonary embolism may be achieved by administering 5000 units of subcutaneous heparin every 8–12 hours and by applying antiembolism stockings, preferably proceeding to full anticoagulation with warfarin.

> **Anticoagulation**
> 5000 Units of heparin subcutaneously every 8-12 hours and antiembolism stockings
> If there are no medical contraindications then proceed to full anticoagulation with warfarin

Care of the joints and limbs

- Daily passive movement of joints
- Splints for hands of tetraplegic patients
- Early internal fixation of limb fractures often required

The joints must be passively moved through the full range each day to prevent stiffness and contractures in those joints that may later recover function and to prevent contractures in other joints, which might also interfere with rehabilitation. Splints to keep the tetraplegic hand in the position of function are particularly important. Early internal fixation of limb fractures is often indicated to assist nursing, particularly as pressure sores in anaesthetic areas may develop unnoticed in plaster casts.

Use of steroids and antibiotics

Use of antibiotics
- Treat only established infections
- Avoid emergence of resistant organisms, particularly in respiratory and urinary tracts

Antibiotics are not normally indicated for the prevention of either urinary or pulmonary infection.

Although an American study has suggested that a short course of high dose methylprednisolone, started within the first eight hours after injury, improves neurological outcome, this has not yet been universally accepted. Indeed, the risk of gastrointestinal stress ulceration is increased by treatment with steroids.

Transfer to a spinal injuries unit

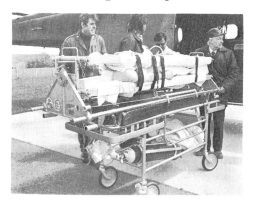

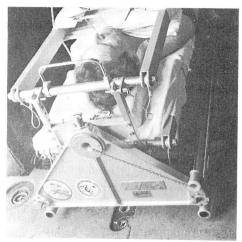

As there are only 11 spinal injuries units in the United Kingdom, most patients will be admitted to a district general hospital for their initial treatment. As soon as spinal cord injury is diagnosed or suspected the nearest spinal injuries unit should be contacted. Immediate transfer is ideal, but this will depend on the general condition of the patient and also on the intensive care facilities available. Unfortunately, some patients will not be fit enough for immediate transfer because of multiple injuries or severe respiratory impairment. In such cases it is advisable to consult, and perhaps arrange a visit by, a spinal injuries consultant.

Transfer to a spinal injuries centre is most easily accomplished by means of a Stryker frame, which can be fitted with a constant tension device for skull traction. The RAF pattern turning frame is similarly equipped and has been specifically developed for use in air evacuation. Tetraplegic patients should be accompanied by a suitably experienced doctor, preferably an anaesthetist, who can quickly intubate the patient if severe respiratory difficulty ensues. Transfer by helicopter is often the ideal and is advisable if the patient has to travel a long distance. In Switzerland immediate helicopter transfer from the site of the accident to a national spinal injuries unit has been associated with an 80% reduction in overall mortality.

Top: this patient was transferred by helicopter to the Duke of Cornwall Spinal Treatment Centre using an RAF pattern turning frame. Below: the constant tension device.

MEDICAL MANAGEMENT IN THE SPINAL INJURIES UNIT

David Grundy, Anthony Tromans

The cervical spine

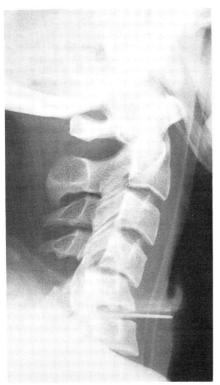

In injuries of the cervical spine skull traction is normally maintained for six weeks initially. The spine may be positioned in flexion, extension, or neutral depending on the nature of the injury. Thus flexion injuries with suspected or obvious damage to the posterior ligamentous complex are treated by placing the neck in a degree of extension. The standard site of insertion of skull calipers need not be changed to achieve this; extension is achieved by correctly positioning a pillow or support under the shoulders. A support under the head produces flexion. Most injuries are managed with the neck in the neutral position. An appropriately sized neck roll is also inserted to maintain normal cervical lordosis.

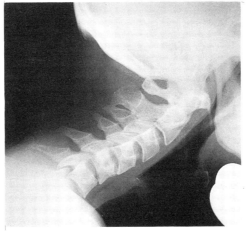

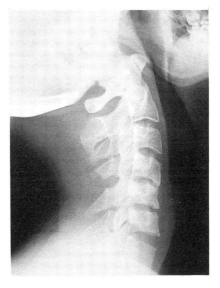

Left: unstable flexion injury in a man who sustained complete tetraplegia below C5. Note forward slip of C4 on C5 and widened interspinous gap, indicating posterior ligamentous damage. Middle and right: the same patient six months later conservatively treated. Flexion-extension views show no appreciable movement but a persisting slight flexion deformity at the site of the previous instability.

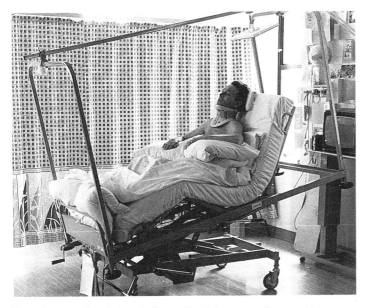

Tetraplegic patient injured after a dive into the shallow end of a swimming pool—profiling before mobilisation into a wheelchair.

Radiographs are taken regularly for position and at six weeks for evidence of bony union, with traction being continued for a further two to three weeks if there are any signs of instability. After traction has been stopped the patient is sat up in bed gradually during the course of a few days, wearing a firm cervical support such as a Philadelphia collar, before being mobilised into a wheelchair. This process is most conveniently achieved using a profiling bed, but the skin over the natal cleft and other pressure areas must be inspected frequently for signs of pressure or shearing. Some patients, specially those with high level lesions, often have postural hypotension at first, so profiling must not be hurried.

If postural hypotension occurs antiembolism stockings and an abdominal binder to reduce the peripheral pooling of blood due to sympathetic paralysis are helpful. Ephedrine 15-30 mg given 20 minutes before profiling starts is also effective. Once the spine is stable the firm collar can often be dispensed with at about 12 weeks after injury and a soft collar worn temporarily for comfort.

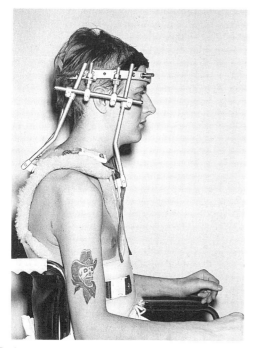

Patient with C6-7 dislocation and incomplete tetraplegia. The dislocation was reduced operatively and posterior spinal fusion performed. The halo was applied and traction administered. Ten days later halo bracing was assembled and the patient was mobilised into a wheelchair.

The application of a halo brace is a useful alternative to skull traction in many patients, once the neck is reduced. It provides stability and allows early mobilisation. Its use is often necessary for up to 12 weeks, when it can be replaced by a soft collar.

Twelve weeks after injury flexion-extension radiographs should be taken under medical supervision if there is any likelihood of instability, but if pain or paraesthesiae occurs the procedure must be discontinued. Most unstable injuries in the lower cervical spine are due to flexion-rotation forces and in the upper cervical spine to hyperextension. If internal fixation is indicated a posterior approach is still the one most often used, but with improvements in modern internal fixation techniques anterior surgery is gaining acceptance.

The decision to perform spinal fusion is usually taken early, and sometimes it will have been performed in the district general hospital before transfer to the spinal injuries unit. The decision about when to operate will depend on the expertise and facilities available and the condition of the patient. However, some patients require late spinal fusion because of failed conservative treatment.

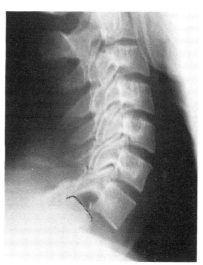 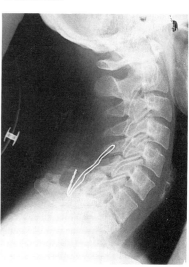

C7-T1 bilateral facet fracture-dislocation with fractures of spinous processes of C6 and C7 and complete tetraplegia below C7. Treated by operative reduction and stabilisation by wiring the spinous processes of C5 to T1 and bone grafting.

Upper cervical spine and cervicothoracic junction

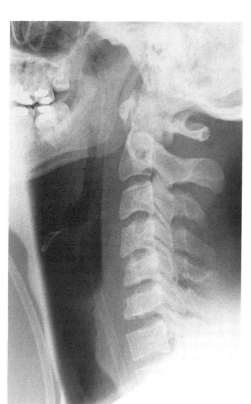

As injuries of the upper cervical spine are often initially associated with acute respiratory failure, prompt appropriate treatment is important, including ventilation if necessary. Other patients may have little or no neurological deficit but again prompt treatment is important to prevent neurological deterioration.

Fractures of the atlas are of two types. The most common, a fracture of the posterior arch, is due to an extension-compression force and is a stable injury which can be safely treated by immobilisation in a firm collar. The second type, the Jefferson fracture, is due to a vertical compression force to the vertex of the skull, resulting in the occipital condyles being driven downwards to produce a bursting injury, in which there is outward displacement of the lateral masses of the atlas and in which the transverse ligament may also have been ruptured. This is an unstable injury with the potential for atlantoxial dislocation, and immobilisation is necessary for at least eight weeks.

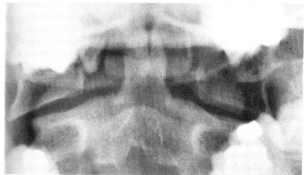

Lateral view (far left): diving injury with compression fractures of the bodies of C5 and C6 and an associated Jefferson fracture of the atlas, not obvious on this view. Anteroposterior view (left) shows Jefferson fracture clearly, with outward displacement of the right lateral mass of the atlas.

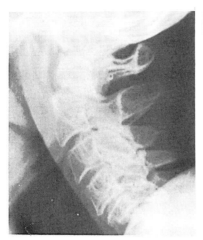
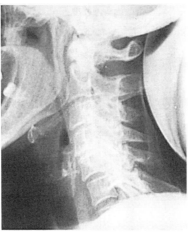

Odontoid fracture in a 64 year old woman, due to hyperextension injury after a fall on to her face at home. It was reduced by applying 4 kg traction force, with atlanto-occipital flexion; the position was subsequently maintained by using a reduced weight of 1·5 kg.

Fractures of the odontoid, usually caused by hyperextension, result in posterior displacement of the odontoid and posterior subluxation of C1 on C2; flexion injuries produce anterior displacement of the odontoid and anterior subluxation of C1 on C2. If displacement is considerable, reduction is achieved by gentle controlled skull traction under radiographic control. Immobiliation is continued for at least three to four months, depending on radiographic signs of healing. Halo bracing is very useful in managing this fracture. Posterior atlantoaxial fusion is necessary if there is non-union and atlantoaxial instability.

The "hangman's" fracture, a traumatic spondylolisthesis of the axis, so called because the bony damage is similar to that seen in judicial hanging, is produced by extension of the head on the neck with distraction. This results in a fracture through the pedicles of the axis in the region of the pars interarticularis, with an anterior slip of the C2 vertebral body on that of C3. Bony union occurs readily, but gentle skull traction should be maintained for six weeks, followed by immobilisation in a firm collar for a further two months. Great care must be taken to avoid overdistraction in this injury. Indeed, in all upper cervical fracture-dislocations control can usually be obtained by reducing the traction force to only 1 to 2 kg once reduction has been achieved. If more weight is used, neurological deterioration may result from overdistraction at the site of injury. An alternative approach when there is no bony displacement or when reduction has been achieved is to apply a halo brace. This avoids overdistraction from skull traction.

The cervicothoracic junction—Closed reduction of a C7-T1 facet dislocation is often difficult if not impossible, in which case operative reduction by facetectomy and posterior fusion is indicated, particularly in patients with an incomplete spinal cord lesion.

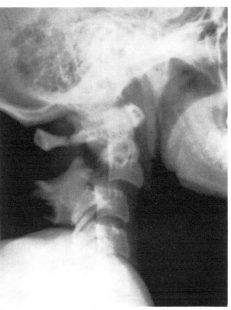

Forced extension injury sustained in car accident by 22 year old woman, resulting in a "hangman's" fracture. There is also associated fracture of posterior arch of atlas.

The thoracolumbar spine

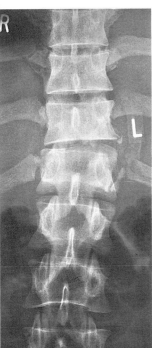
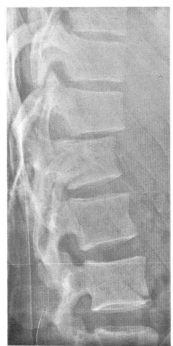
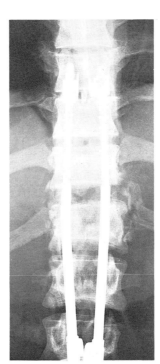
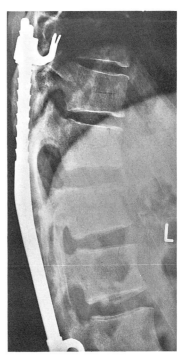

A 29 year old motorcyclist with complete paraplegia below T11 as a result of a fracture-dislocation of T11-T12. Normal alignment was achieved by using Harrington rods. Note the normal thoracolumbar curve preserved by shaping the rods.

Medical management in spinal injuries unit

Most patients with thoracolumbar injuries can be managed conservatively with an initial period of bed rest for eight to 12 weeks followed by gradual mobilisation in a spinal brace. If there is gross deformity or if the injury is unstable, especially if the spinal cord injury is incomplete, operative reduction, surgical instrumentation, and bone grafting correct the deformity and permit early mobilisation.

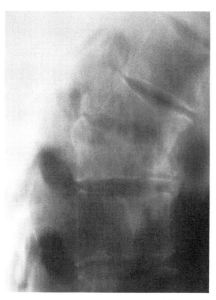
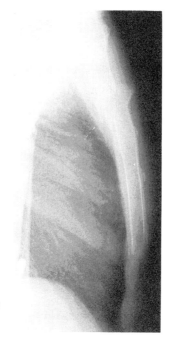

Wedge compression fractures of T5 and T6 in association with a fracture of the sternum.

Laminectomy has no place because it may render the spine unstable and does not achieve adequate decompression of the spinal cord except in the rare instance of a depressed fracture of a lamina. If decompression is felt to be desirable, surgery should be aimed at the site of bony compression, which is generally anteriorly. An anterior approach with vertebrectomy by an experienced surgeon carries little added morbidity.

Before a patient with an unstable injury is mobilised, the spine is braced, the brace remaining in place until bony union occurs. Even if operative reduction has been undertaken, bracing may still be required for up to six months, depending on the type of spinal fusion performed. Injuries to the upper thoracic spine are sometimes associated with a fracture of the sternum, which makes a stable injury unstable because of the loss of the normal anterior splinting effect of the sternum. It is very difficult to brace the upper thoracic spine, and if such a patient is mobilised too quickly a severe flexion deformity of the spine may develop.

Pulmonary embolism, para-articular heterotopic ossification, spasticity, and contractures

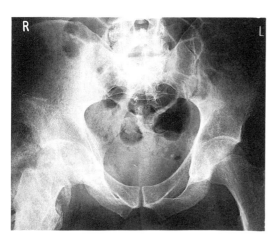

Heterotopic ossification in the right hip.

Factors that aggravate spasticity

- Pressure sores
- Contractures
- Urinary tract infection or calculus
- Anal fissure
- Infected ingrowing toenail
- Fracture

Pulmonary embolism—Anticoagulation, which in the absence of contraindications should have been started 24 to 36 hours after the accident, is continued throughout the initial period of bed rest until the patient is fully mobile in a wheelchair. If pulmonary embolism does occur the management is as for non-paralysed patients.

Para-articular heterotopic ossification—After injury to the spinal cord new bone is often laid down in the soft tissues around paralysed joints, particularly the hip and knee. The cause is unknown, although local trauma has been suggested. It usually presents with erythema, induration, or swelling near a joint. There is pronounced osteoblastic activity, but the new bone formed does not mature for at least 18 months. This has an important bearing on treatment in that if excision of heterotopic bone is required because of gross restriction of movement or bony ankylosis of a joint, surgery must be delayed for at least 18 months—until the new bone is mature. Earlier surgical intervention may provoke further new bone formation, thus compounding the original condition. As yet there is no convincing evidence that treatment with disodium etidronate or non-steroidal anti-inflammatory drugs prevents the progression of this complication.

Spasticity—Spasticity is seen only in patients with upper motor neurone lesions of the cord whose intact spinal reflex arcs below the level of the lesion are isolated from higher centres. It usually increases in severity during the first few weeks after injury, after the period of spinal shock. In incomplete lesions it is usually more pronounced and can be severe enough to prevent patients with good power in the legs from walking. Patients with severe spasticity and imbalance of opposing muscle groups have a tendency to develop contractures. It is important to realise that once a contracture occurs spasticity is increased and a vicious circle is established with further deformity resulting. Although excessive spasticity may hamper patients' activities or even throw them out of their wheelchairs or make walking impossible, spasticity may have advantages. It maintains muscle bulk, decreases osteoporosis, and improves venous return.

Treatment of severe spasticity is initially directed at removing any

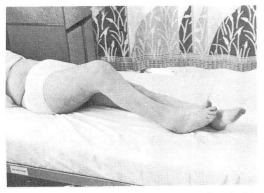

Contractures at right hip and knee, associated with unrelieved spasticity.

obvious precipitating cause. An irritative lesion in the paralysed part, such as a pressure sore, urinary tract infection or calculus, anal fissure, infected ingrowing toenail, or fracture, tends to increase spasticity. Passive stretching of spastic muscles and regular standing are helpful in relieving spasticity and preventing contractures. The drugs most commonly used to decrease spasticity are baclofen, which acts at spinal level, and dantrolene sodium, which acts direct on skeletal muscle. Although diazepam relieves spasticity, its sedative action and habit forming tendency limit its usefulness. If spasticity is localised it can be relieved by interrupting the nerve supply to the muscles affected by neurectomy after a diagnostic block using a long acting local anaesthetic (bupivacaine). For example, in patients with severe hip adductor spasticity obturator neurectomy is effective. Alternatively, motor point injections, initially using bupivacaine, followed by either 6% aqueous phenol or 45% ethyl alcohol for a more lasting effect, are useful in selected patients. Rarely, and if severe spasticity cannot be otherwise relieved, an intrathecal block with 6% aqueous phenol or absolute alcohol is indicated. The effect of phenol usually lasts a few months, that of alcohol is permanent. The main disadvantage in the use of either is that they convert an upper motor to a lower motor neurone lesion, and thus affect bladder, bowel, and sexual function. The use of intrathecal baclofen administered by an implanted reservoir and pump is gaining acceptance in the treatment of patients with severe spasticity and avoids the drawbacks of the above destructive procedures. The strength and frequency of administration can be adjusted to give an acceptable level of spasticity.

Contractures—A contracture may be a result of immobilisation, spasticity, or muscle imbalance between opposing muscle groups. It may respond to conservative measures such as gradual stretching of affected muscles, often with the use of splints. If these measures fail to correct the deformity or are inappropriate, then surgical correction by tenotomy, tendon lengthening, or muscle division may be required. For example, a flexion contracture of the hip responds to an iliopsoas myotomy with division of the anterior capsule and soft tissues over the front of the joint.

Pressure sores

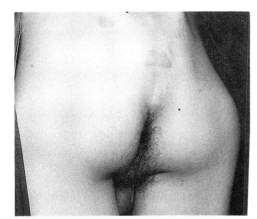

Pressure marks over sacrum and left posterior iliac crest. Relief of pressure over these areas must be continued until marks have faded. In this patient this was achieved only after three days of bed rest with appropriate positioning.

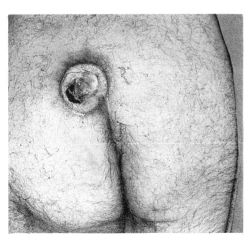

Effect of unrelieved pressure—a deep sacral pressure sore.

Pressure sores form as a result of ischaemia, caused by unrelieved pressure, particularly over bony prominences. They may affect not only the skin but also subcutaneous fat, muscle, and deeper structures. If near a joint, septic arthritis may supervene. The commonest sites are over the ischial tuberosity, greater trochanter, and sacrum. Pressure sores are a major cause of readmission to hospital, yet they are wholly preventable by vigilance and recognition of simple principles.

Regular changes of position in bed every two to three hours and lifting in the wheelchair every 15 minutes are essential. A suitable mattress and wheelchair cushion are particularly important. The cushion should be selected for the individual patient after measuring the interface pressures between the ischial tuberosities and the cushion. Cushions need frequent checking and renewing if necessary. Shearing forces to the skin from underlying structures are avoided by correct lifting; the skin should never be dragged along supporting surfaces. Patients must not lie for long periods with the skin unprotected on X ray diagnostic units or on operating tables (in this situation Roho mattress sections placed under the patient are of benefit). A pressure clinic is extremely useful in checking the sitting posture, assessing the wheelchair and cushion, and generally instilling pressure consciousness into patients. If a red mark on the skin is noticed which does not fade within 20 minutes the patient should avoid all pressure on that area until the redness and any underlying induration disappears.

If an established sore is present, any slough is excised and the wound is dressed, using a desloughing agent if necessary. Once the wound is clean and has healthy granulation tissue, normal saline dressings may be used. Complete relief of pressure on the affected area is essential until healing has occurred. Indications for surgery are: (a) a large sore which would take too long to heal using conservative methods; (b) a sore with infected bone in its base; (c) a discharging sinus with an underlying bursa. If possible, surgical treatment is by excision of the sore and any underlying bony prominence, with direct closure in layers, leaving a small linear scar. Most pressure sores can be managed in this way. Recurrence is uncommon and if it occurs can be more easily treated after this type of surgery than if large areas of tissues have been disturbed by previous use of a flap.

UROLOGICAL MANAGEMENT

David Grundy, John Cumming

In 1917 Thomson-Walker stated that almost half of all patients with spinal cord injury died of urinary sepsis within two months, and the total death rate from urinary sepsis was 80%. Despite vastly improved management, urinary tract complications are still the main cause of morbidity and mortality. In recent years clinicians have put more emphasis on achieving continence if at all possible, but the main aim remains the preservation of renal function.

> **Aims of bladder management**
> Preservation of renal function
> Continence

Early management

> **Intermittent urethral catheterisation**
> * Strictly aseptic technique
> * Catheterise 6 hourly initially (12 Ch or 14 Ch Nelaton catheter)
> * Restrict fluids until voiding occurs
> * Treat significant urinary tract infection

Intermittent urethral catheterisation

Once the patient is in a spinal injuries unit the standard method of bladder drainage in the first few weeks is by intermittent urethral catheterisation with a 12 Ch or 14 Ch Nelaton catheter, using a strictly aseptic technique. This is normally undertaken by a trained nursing team. The fluid intake should be restricted so that the urinary output is no more than 1500 ml/24 hours until the patient starts voiding. At this stage the fluid intake can be increased. Catheterisation should be repeated regularly, usually every six hours at first, to prevent overdistention of the bladder. The aim is to have a volume of less than 500 ml at each catheterisation.

The urine is cultured weekly and at other times if indicated; infection that produces systemic effects or $>10^8$ organisms/1 or >50 white blood cells/high power field is treated with the appropriate antibacterial drug. It is particularly important to eradicate infection with *Proteus* sp, a urea splitting organism, as it is associated with the highest incidence of calculi; these calculi, composed of calcium phosphate and magnesium ammonium phosphate, readily form in infected alkaline urine.

After the period of spinal shock, involuntary reflex detrusor activity (detrusor hyperreflexia) is seen in most patients with a suprasacral cord lesion. Patients who may later be able to manage their bladders by self intermittent catheterisation (see below) should be catheterised every six hours but no attempt made to empty the bladder beforehand. In other patients the suprapubic area is tapped to induce a detrusor contraction, and this is continued until urinary flow ceases. Suprapubic abdominal compression is then immediately performed to ensure that the bladder is empty (tapping and expression).

When male patients begin to void they wear condoms attached to urinary drainage bags but still continue intermittent catheterisation. The fluid intake is increased, and as the volume of residual urine at each catheterisation falls the frequency of catheterisation is reduced. When the daily residual urine is less than 100 ml on three consecutive occasions catheterisation can be discontinued. At this stage, usually about 6–12 weeks after injury, bladder training is complete—that is, effective emptying of the bladder has been achieved. Patients continue to wear condoms attached to urinary draining bags and are instructed to continue to tap and express the bladder every two to three hours throughout the day. If poor bladder emptying is suspected later, measuring residual urine by abdominal ultrasound scan is useful.

Suprapubic catheterisation

Suprapubic catheterisation using a 10 Ch or 15 Ch catheter is increasingly used as a method of bladder drainage in the first few weeks after spinal cord injury. It avoids urethral instrumentation, with its risks of periurethral abscess, urethral diverticulum, fistula formation, and epididymo-orchitis, and permits a high fluid intake of at least 3 litres every 24 hours. However, its use is not entirely trouble free, and the catheter can block with calcareous deposits.

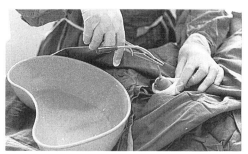

Intermittent urethral catheterisation.

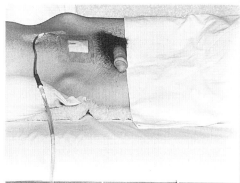

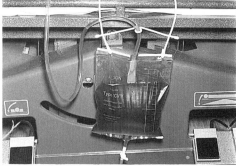

A 15 Ch suprapubic catheter in situ, with sealed drainage system.

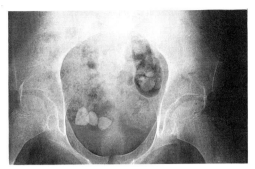

Bladder calculi associated with use of indwelling urethral catheter.

Optimum requirements for self intermittent catheterisation

- Absent or minimal detrusor activity
- Large bladder capacity
- Adequate bladder outlet resistance
- Sufficient manual dexterity
- Pain free catheterisation
- Patient motivation

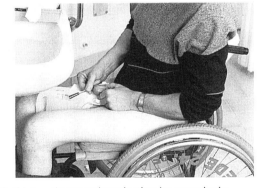

Self intermittent catheterisation by paraplegic patient.

Investigations using:

Serum creatinine

Urine culture

Residual urine

Intravenous urogram

Renal ultrasound scan and plain abdominal radiograph

Renogram

Videourodynamics $\begin{cases} \text{cystometrogram} \\ \text{cystourethrogram} \end{cases}$

Indwelling urethral catheterisation

If the urine is already infected when the patient is admitted to the spinal injuries unit it is preferable to continue with an indwelling urethral catheter until the urine is cleared of infection and debris, when intermittent urethral catheterisation can be started. If the patient has been transferred after two to three weeks it is wiser to continue with an indwelling catheter until six weeks after injury. The long term use of an indwelling urethral catheter, however, can lead to urethral damage in both men and women. In women with contractile neuropathic bladders, the strong detrusor contractions can expel both balloon and catheter and cause dilatation of the urethra. This forced dilatation can leave the urethra with a calibre to rival that of the vagina. In men, the catheter can cause pressure necrosis of the urethra, which may lead to an ever increasing hypospadias and eventually a completely open penile urethra.

A 12 Ch or 14 Ch Foley catheter with a 5-10 ml balloon should be used. A latex catheter should be changed weekly, but a silicone catheter, which is preferable, may be retained for up to six weeks, at which stage bladder training is usually started. Long term urethral catheterisation is the method of choice in many women with tetraplegia and in older patients. As patients with indwelling urethral catheters are prone to develop calculi, a weekly or twice weekly bladder washout with Suby-G solution is recommended. Repeated episodes of blocked catheter should be investigated by cystoscopy and, if present, calculi should be crushed and evacuated with an Ellik evacuator. The urine will inevitably become colonised with bacteria, but antibiotics are not normally used unless the patient develops systemic signs of infection.

Self intermittent catheterisation

When intermittent catheterisation has been performed by the nursing staff, self intermittent catheterisation (SIC) can start as soon as patients begin to sit up. Patients catheterise themselves with the aim of remaining continent between catheterisations and therefore avoiding the need to wear urinary drainage apparatuses. A 12 Ch or 14 Ch Nelaton catheter or, in some women, a silver catheter, is used. It may be possible to decide at an early stage after injury that self intermittent catheterisation is likely to be the method of choice for long term bladder management, and in these patients fluid restriction may not be appropriate. Indeed, ideally a large capacity bladder is useful so that the number of catheterisations can be kept to a minimum, usually four to five in 24 hours.

Self intermittent catheterisation is particularly applicable to patients with a non-contractile detrusor, usually associated with injury to the conus medullaris or cauda equina, for whom it is the most satisfactory method of bladder management.

Even if reflex detrusor activity is present self intermittent catheterisation may be successful, although anticholinergic drugs such as propantheline, oxybutynin, and imipramine may help to reduce detrusor activity; imipramine also increases bladder outlet resistance. Self intermittent catheterisation is especially suitable for women, as a satisfactory urine collecting device is not available. As far as the incidence of infection, development of calculi, and renal function are concerned, the long term results of self intermittent catheterisation are excellent and compare favourably with those of other methods of bladder management.

Investigations

Measurement of the serum creatinine concentration, culture of urine, and estimation of residual urine (using abdominal ultrasound scans when appropriate) are performed regularly. Intravenous urography is performed initially about three months after the injury to give baseline information about the urinary tract, although even at this early stage fullness or early dilatation of the pelvicalyceal system and ureters due to bladder outlet obstruction is occasionally seen.

Urological management

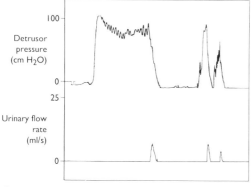

Cystometrogram recording shown high pressure contractions in a contractile neurophatic bladder. Note that the urine is passed when the bladder and distal sphincter are beginning to relax, showing the characteristic pattern of detrusor-sphincter dyssynergia.

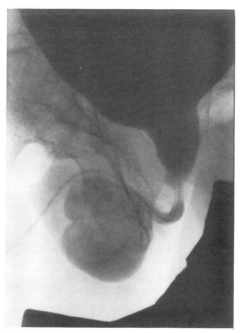

Cystourethrogram during micturition showing a wide open bladder neck and obstruction at the level of the distal urethral sphincter. Large urethral diverticulum is also shown.

Later management

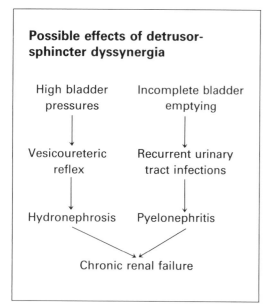

Possible effects of detrusor-sphincter dyssynergia

Further investigation with renal ultrasound scanning and plain abdominal radiography is repeated at intervals, within a few months or a year at first but, if bladder emptying remains satisfactory and the patient is asymptomatic, yearly review is normally advised and in some patients, particularly women, it can be increased to up to three yearly. Lifelong urological follow up is still essential, however, as late bladder outlet obstruction and other complications such as calculi may occur. It must be remembered that, because of absent sensation, renal and ureteric calculi may be asymptomatic. If the patient has had adverse reactions to contrast media, renography is safer than intravenous urography.

Videourodynamics should be performed to plan future management of the bladder and distal urethral sphincter. A baseline videourodynamic investigation is performed after intravenous urography and consists of a study of the relation of pressure to volume of the bladder during slow filling and voiding (shown on a cystometrogram), combined with radiographic screening of the bladder and urethra during both the filling and the voiding phases of micturition. The state of the detrusor and sphincter muscle activity is shown, and detrusor-sphincter dyssynergia (see below), other causes of bladder outlet obstruction, and vesicoureteric reflux may be seen.

In normal voiding a detrusor contraction is accompanied by an active relaxation of the distal urethral sphincter; the detrusor and sphincter work synergically. However, in many patients with a suprasacral cord lesion the distal urethral sphincter actively contracts during a detrusor contraction; this is detrusor-sphincter dyssynergia. Subsequently both detrusor and sphincter relax and urine is passed. However, the detrusor contraction fades away quite rapidly and before the bladder has emptied. It is the failure of the continued detrusor contraction, rather than bladder outflow obstruction, that results in the urine residue. This residue encourages recurrent urinary tract infections, and the high intravesical pressures can lead to vesicoureteric reflux, hydronephrosis, pyelonephritis, and stone formation. If videourodynamics is performed early detrusor-sphincter dyssynergia can be detected before damage occurs.

After the initial investigations, bladder management may be modified as necessary. The possible options should be discussed with the patient. The aims are to preserve renal function and if possible achieve urinary continence.

The introduction of self intermittent catheterisation has enabled these aims to be met in an increasing number of patients, both men and women, particularly in those with acontractile bladders, and the method is on the whole preferred by patients. In hospital a new catheter is used for each catheterisation, but at home the method becomes a clean though not necessarily sterile technique, and a catheter can be reused several times.

Despite satisfactory bladder emptying, some patients suffer recurrent urinary tract infections, for which acidifying the urine (using a non-effervescent ascorbic acid preparation) or using a urinary antiseptic (such as hexamine) may be beneficial. Specific antibacterial treatment should only be used in patients with systemic signs of infection. Whenever possible a high urinary output of at least 3 litres/ 24 hours also helps to minimise infection.

There is little place for urinary diversion procedures, such as creating an ileal conduit, in patients with spinal cord injuries because the ileal segment causes back pressure on the upper renal tract. This is particularly relevant to patients whose life expectancy is more than 10 years.

Men

Acontractile bladders in men are usually the result of low spinal cord injuries, which preserve hand function, and are therefore best managed by self catheterisation. Episodes of incontinence may reflect a reduced bladder outflow resistance, which can be modified pharmacologically with imipramine or phenylpropanolamine.

Bladders of incontinent men are usually of the contractile neuropathic type, often with high intravesical pressures, detrusor-sphincter dyssynergia, intermittent uncontrolled voids, and reduced bladder capacities. Some will respond to suprapubic "tapping" to stimulate a contraction with voiding and, if bladder compliance and capacity allow, these patients can be managed with condom drainage. About a third of patients with suprasacral cord lesions and reflex bladder emptying, however, require an endoscopic distal sphincterotomy. A single incision through the full depth and along the full length of the distal sphincter is sufficient to relieve the obstruction caused by the sphincter. Some contractile bladders fail to resume their activity after this procedure, and it may take weeks or months for the contractions to return.

Retaining a condom on the penis is difficult for men whose abdomen overflows the pubic area and whose penis retracts within the pubic fat. Implanting rigid or semirigid penile prostheses not only helps retain the condom for urine collection but also can be used for sexual purposes.

An alternative to distal sphincterotomy and condom drainage is bladder augmentation with an ileocystoplasty to allow sufficient capacity for satisfactory self intermittent catheterisation. Although this requires a more extensive operation, it has the effect of increasing bladder capacity to 600-1000 ml or more and lowering the intravesical pressure. Most men become continent between self intermittent catheterisations, although this cannot be guaranteed.

Bladder neck obstruction is rare but, if present, may be useful in maintaining continence when the patient is being managed by self intermittent catheterisation. Although self intermittent catheterisation is so successful, in some patients with an acontractile bladder and an incompetent urethral closure mechanism, emptying is best achieved by abdominal straining or suprapubic compression. Condom drainage is often necessary when the patient leaks urine between acts of voiding. If bladder emptying is unsatisfactory in these patients it is likely to be due to an isolated distal sphincter obstruction that requires sphincterotomy. Rarely, bladder neck obstruction is the cause, and bladder neck incision may be needed to reduce outflow resistance. Reducing outflow resistance may be achieved by an α adrenergic blocking drug such as prazosin. A minority of male patients refuse to try self intermittent catheterisation, feeling that condom drainage will be less troublesome. If self intermittent catheterisation is not possible because of insufficient hand function or if the patient, after several weeks' trial, cannot stay dry between catheterisations, the bladder should be managed by condom drainage. In practice, most men are still managed by this method.

As patients are surviving much longer than before, prostatic obstruction requiring transurethral prostatectomy is becoming more common. Long term management using a Foley catheter may be indicated for elderly or frail patients.

Long term prevention of urinary tract infection

- High fluid intake if possible
- Ensure effective bladder emptying
- (Acidification of urine)
- (Administration of urinary antiseptics)

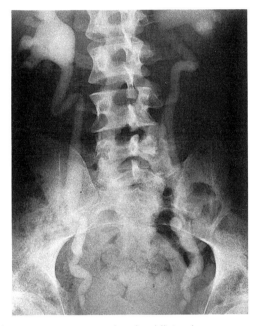

Intravenous urogram showing bilateral hydronephrosis resulting from detrusor-sphincter dyssynergia. Treated by distal sphincterotomy with subsequent resolution of hydronephrosis.

Drugs used to manage the neuropathic bladder

Action	Drug
To increase detrusor activity	Carbachol, bethanechol orally, distigmine bromide intramuscularly
To reduce detrusor activity	Propantheline, oxybutynin, imipramine orally
To increase bladder outflow resistance	Imipramine, phenylpropanolamine orally
To reduce bladder outflow resistance	Prazosin orally, phentolamine intravenously or intramuscularly

---

Female patients

- Satisfactory urine collecting device not available
- Greater emphasis on self intermittent catheterisation, or indwelling catheter in tetraplegic women
- Bladder function commonly disturbed during menstruation and pregnancy
- Renal failure rare

Autonomic dysreflexia

Pounding headache

Profuse sweating

Flushing or blotchiness above level of lesion

Danger—intracranial haemorrhage

Treatment of autonomic dysreflexia

Remove the cause

Sit patient up

Treat with:

    Nifedipine 5-10 mg sublingually
    or

    Glyceryl trinitrate 250 μg sublingually
    or

    Phentolamine 5-10 mg intravenously

Spinal or epidural anaesthetic (rarely)

Distal sphincterotomy (at a later stage)

Women

In women there is no place for bladder neck incision or sphincterotomy and the results of bladder augmentation by cystoplasty are perhaps not sufficiently predictable to be reliably beneficial.

Until recently the standard method of bladder emptying for women was for the patient to transfer on to the toilet, usually every two to four hours, and tap and express the bladder if there was reflex detrusor activity or express alone if the bladder was acontractile. Though the method is still advocated, patients often remain wet between acts of voiding and have to wear incontinence pads, and therefore self intermittent catheterisation is preferable. If a woman is still incontinent between self catheterisations then an indwelling catheter should be considered. Tetraplegic women with insufficient hand function to perform self catheterisation should be offered an indwelling Foley catheter as it can revolutionise a patient's quality of life. As in men, this is also applicable to elderly or frail patients and others who cannot remain continent.

However, indwelling catheters have their own particular problems. Recurrent blockage of the catheter due to phosphates or deposits in infected urine can be difficult to treat despite bladder washouts and changes of catheter. The use of antibiotics should be resisted unless there are signs of systemic infection. Cystoscopy and washout of the bladder with an Ellik evacuator are often useful to remove all infected debris, stone fragments, and infected urine. Contractile neuropathic bladders have a tendency to bypass the catheter and even to expel catheters with the balloon inflated. The temptation to increase the balloon capacity should be resisted, otherwise the urethra will become dilated and traumatised, making correction of the problem difficult. The bladder neck and urethra can be tightened with a Stamey colposuspension. This relies on two nylon slings inserted on either side of the urethra at the bladder neck. These are passed from suprapubic incisions and suspend the vagina and paravaginal tissues from the abdominal wall. If this is ineffective a Feneley procedure is necessary. In this operation, the urethra is invaginated into the bladder and closed with a suture. A suprapubic catheter drains the bladder.

Autonomic dysreflexia

Autonomic dysreflexia is seen particularly in patients with cervical cord injuries above the sympathetic outflow but may also occur in those with high thoracic lesions above T6. It may occur at any time after the period of spinal shock and is usually due to a distended bladder caused by a blocked catheter, or to poor bladder emptying as a result of detrusor-sphincter dyssynergia. The distension of the bladder results in reflex sympathetic overactivity below the level of the spinal cord lesion, causing vasoconstriction and systemic hypertension. The carotid and aortic baroreceptors are stimulated and respond via the vasomotor centre with increased vagal tone and resulting bradycardia; but the peripheral vasodilation that would normally have relieved the hypertension does not occur because stimuli cannot pass distally through the injured cord. Characteristically the patient suffers a pounding headache, profuse sweating, and flushing or blotchiness of the skin above the level of the spinal cord lesion. Without prompt treatment, intracranial haemorrhage may occur.

Other conditions in which visceral stimulation can result in autonomic dysreflexia include urinary tract infection, bladder calculi, a loaded colon, an anal fissure, ejaculation during sexual intercourse, and labour.

Treatment consists of removing the precipitating cause. If this lies in the urinary tract catheterisation is often necessary. If hypertension persists nifedipine 5-10 mg sublingually, glyceryl trinitrate 250 μg sublingually, or phentolamine 5-10 mg intravenously is given. If inadequately treated the patient can become sensitised and develop repeated attacks with minimal stimuli. Occasionally the sympathetic reflex activity may have to be blocked by a spinal or epidural anaesthetic. Later management may include a sphincterotomy if detrusor-sphincter dyssynergia is causing the symptoms; performed under spinal anaesthesia, the risk of autonomic dysreflexia is lessened.

Long term bladder management (methods in parentheses less satisfactory)

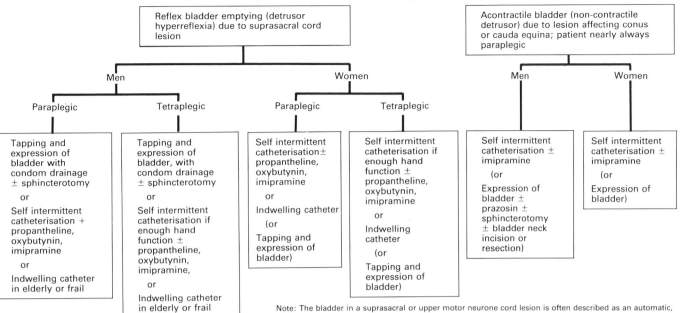

Reflex bladder emptying (detrusor hyperreflexia) due to suprasacral cord lesion				Acontractile bladder (non-contractile detrusor) due to lesion affecting conus or cauda equina; patient nearly always paraplegic	
Men		**Women**		**Men**	**Women**
Paraplegic	Tetraplegic	Paraplegic	Tetraplegic		
Tapping and expression of bladder with condom drainage ± sphincterotomy or Self intermittent catheterisation + propantheline, oxybutynin, imipramine or Indwelling catheter in elderly or frail	Tapping and expression of bladder, with condom drainage ± sphincterotomy or Self intermittent catheterisation if enough hand function ± propantheline, oxybutynin, imipramine, or Indwelling catheter in elderly or frail	Self intermittent catheterisation± propantheline, oxybutynin, imipramine or Indwelling catheter (or Tapping and expression of bladder)	Self intermittent catheterisation if enough hand function ± propantheline, oxybutynin, imipramine or Indwelling catheter (or Tapping and expression of bladder)	Self intermittent catheterisation ± imipramine (or Expression of bladder ± prazosin ± sphincterotomy ± bladder neck incision or resection)	Self intermittent catheterisation ± imipramine (or Expression of bladder)

Note: The bladder in a suprasacral or upper motor neurone cord lesion is often described as an automatic, reflex, or upper motor neurone bladder; in a conus or cauda equina lesion it is often referred to as a flaccid or lower motor neurone bladder. These terms are best avoided.

Other methods of bladder management

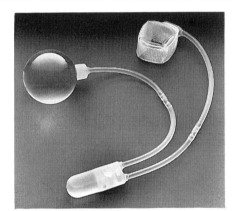

In recent years the artificial urinary sphincter (AUS) has been used increasingly for treating neuropathic incontinence. It can be used for patients with either acontractile or contractile bladders. In contractile bladders augmentation cystoplasty will keep intravesical pressure low and provide greater capacity. The mechanical reliability of the artificial sphincter (AMS800) is satisfactorily high but there is an appreciable risk of infection and erosion. In view of these factors, artificial urinary sphincters are probably best reserved for ambulant spinally injured patients with disturbed bladder and sphincter functions.

Artificial urinary sphincter. Inflatable cuff is normally placed around bladder neck. Control pump, placed in the scrotum in men and in the labium in women, controls the flow of fluid between reservoir (in the prevesical space) and cuff. To void the fluid is transferred from cuff to reservoir.

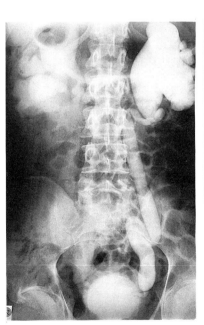 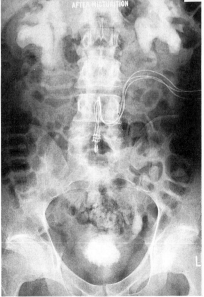

Another recent advance, applicable to some patients with a suprasacral cord lesion, is the sacral anterior nerve root stimulator (SARS), in which the patient has a radiolinked implant to stimulate the S2, S3, and S4 anterior nerve roots. By activating the implant the patient can empty the bladder at will, reduce the residual volume, and possibly achieve continence. The implant can also assist in defecation and in obtaining an (implant-driven) erection in some male patients. Because the posterior sacral roots are also divided the procedure is not suitable for patients with an incomplete lesion, as they will lose useful sensation below the level of injury as well as reflex erections.

Left: gross bilateral hydronephrosis and hydroureter, due to detrusor-sphincter dyssynergia, which did not respond to sphincterotomy. Right: hydronephrosis improved as a result of more efficient voiding after implantation of a sacral anterior nerve root stimulator.

NURSING

Catriona Wood, David Grundy

The major objectives in caring for people with spinal cord lesions are to: (a) identify problems and prevent deterioration; (b) prevent secondary complications; (c) facilitate maximum functional recovery for each individual; (d) support patients and their families as they adjust to the patient's changed physical status; (e) be aware of the effect of the injuries on patients' self esteem, giving high priority to establishing a new sense of self worth; (f) educate patients and their relatives in all aspects of care needed to maintain well being.

The organisation of nursing in a spinal injuries unit must recognise that the patient will spend a long time in hospital—probably four to nine months, that most patients are aged 15-35, and that most are men (4:1 men to women). Patients will initially be very dependent on others, and those with high lesions may continue to be dependent and have a disappointing level of neurological recovery.

These factors contribute to establishing close and supportive relationships between staff and patients, which blur boundaries between professional and personal roles. This, with the psychological support required by patients, increases stress for the staff. Good teamwork, a supportive environment, and adequate staffing levels are therefore necessary.

The psychological trauma of spinal cord injury is profound and prolonged. The impact on the injured person and his or her family is highly individual and varies from patient to patient throughout the course of their care. Fear and anxiety, worsened by sensory deprivation, may initially be considerable and may continue in some degree for many months. During the acute phase, particularly when patients are confined to bed, they may experience a wide variety of mood swings including anger, depression, and euphoria. They may exhibit behaviour identifiable with a normal grieving process—guilt, denial—or other coping mechanisms such as regression. They will suffer from a sense of frustration, be verbally demanding, or sometimes withdrawn.

Relatives often progress to adjustment much more quickly than the patients themselves, and this may complicate planning for the future. Intervention must take into consideration the coping mechanisms used by the patients and their families. Long term decisions must not be taken before patients are willing and able to participate.

Certain landmarks in rehabilitation are especially stressful for the patient. Being mobilised from bed to wheelchair is one, with its combination of blood pressure instability, physical exhaustion, and the shock of coming to terms with an altered body image. Any occasion experienced for the first time after injury is likely to be stressful. Most spinal injuries units have an "aids to daily living" (ADL) flat where patients and their relatives can stay before their first weekend at home and where they will be close to help, if necessary. Visits to home and friends are major psychological and physical hurdles, and patients must be prepared for these events and supported through them. Visits should be discussed afterwards, initially with staff from the unit with whom they feel safe, and later with their family and friends. Discharge from hospital is a considerable challenge, with patients and their families having to cope with tiredness, loneliness and isolation, and the changed relationships caused by injury.

Continuing support will be needed for at least two to three years while the patient adjusts to his or her lifestyle and learns to accept it.

Nursing aims

- Identify problems and help prevent deterioration
- Prevent secondary complications
- Maximise functional recovery
- Support patients and relatives
- Maintain patients' self esteem
- Educate patients and relatives

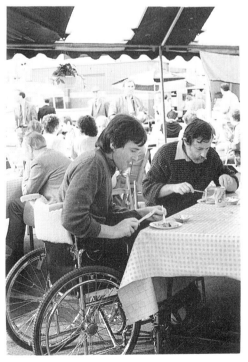

Member of staff and patient enjoying a day away from the unit.

Nursing management

Pressure relief in the accident and emergency department

- Remove all clothing
- Use pressure relieving mattress
- Lift or log roll half hourly
- Examine skin for marking or damage

In the accident and emergency department

A patient with major trauma is normally placed on a trauma trolley with a rigid base in case resuscitation is necessary. The chin lift or jaw thrust manoeuvres, and not head tilt, are used for patients with cervical spine instability if they are not fully conscious.

The spine must be kept straight and never flexed. If the patient is received wearing a hard collar it must remain in place until removed by the doctor. If a cervical spine injury is suspected and no collar has been applied the neck should be immobilised using a semirigid collar taped to sandbags on each side of the head. All clothing should be removed to facilitate full examination and inspection for skin damage. Care should be taken not to extend the arms above head level.

After upper thoracic and cervical cord lesions, patients become poikilothermic, taking on the surrounding temperature, with a tendency to hypothermia. During the assessment phase care must be taken to maintain patients' temperatures within normal levels.

Once a spinal cord injury has been diagnosed, care of the pressure areas is extremely important. If delay in admission to the ward is expected the patient should ideally be transferred to a mattress that will reduce pressure on the bony prominences, and log rolling into the the lateral position is then performed for one minute every half hour.

In the ward

An holistic approach is essential to meet the various problems with which a patient may present. In the initial acute phase, nursing care will be implemented to meet the patient's own inability to maintain his or her own activities of daily living. As the patient progresses, the nurse's role becomes more supportive and educative, with the patient taking responsibility through self care or by directing carers.

Posturing

- Support injured spine in alignment
- Maintain limbs and joints in functional position
- Relieve pressure

Posturing—Regular position changing usually every two to three hours initially, skin inspection (maintaining spinal alignment), and posturing of limbs are essential for a patient with spinal cord injury. The aims are simple: (a) to support the injured spine in a good healing position; (b) to maintain limbs and joints in a functional position, thus avoiding deformity and contractures and reducing the incidence of spasticity; and (c) to relieve pressure. There are several ways of achieving these aims, so the method chosen should suit the patient and the availability and skill of the nursing staff.

Choice of bed—The standard King's Fund bed or profiling bed with a mattress consisting of layers of varying density foam is suitable for most patients and is probably the best bed for tetraplegic patients, facilitating good positioning of the shoulders and arms. It needs a trained turning team of nurses. The Egerton turning and tilting bed is particularly suitable for heavy patients and those with multiple injuries; it permits easier nursing but still requires a trained team and frequent inspection of pressure points and natal cleft. A Stryker frame, in which turning can be managed with fewer staff, is useful for patients undergoing spinal surgery and for the transfer of patients between hospitals.

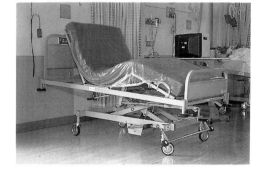

Profiling bed.

Spinal alignment—Before undertaking a turn or preparing to lift a patient, spinal alignment should be maintained by checking (when the patient is supine) that the nose, sternum, and symphysis pubis are in alignment and that the shoulders and hips are level.

Lifts and turns

Straight lifting is used for transferring patients and lifting them to the side of the bed for nursing care. (1) The head nurse holds the neck and head with both hands under the neck and both wrists supporting the patient's head under the ears. (2) The lifters' arms are inserted one at a time, starting at the top of the patient, with counter pressure from the other side to prevent movement of the injured spine. Once the nurses' arms are in position (3) the patient may be lifted (4). After the lift (5) the arms are withdrawn in reverse order, one of the team applying counter pressure by placing her or his arms across the patient.

A log roll is needed for carrying out nursing care and for lateral positioning of both paraplegic and tetraplegic patients. The illustration shows how the paraplegic patient should be held (6). Note that the injury site is well supported, with the lumbar pillow remaining in situ. When the log roll is complete (7) the patient remains supported by pillows, particularly in the lumbar curve. Note also the alignment of the shoulder, hip and iliac crest, and upper leg. A tetraplegic patient will need a head hold but will not require a lumbar pillow.

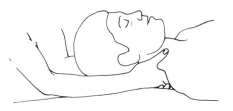

(1) Head hold with head and neck supported by nurse's wrists and hands.

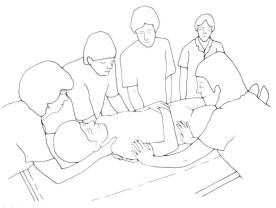

(2) Inserting arms under patient with counter pressure to prevent movement of the spine.

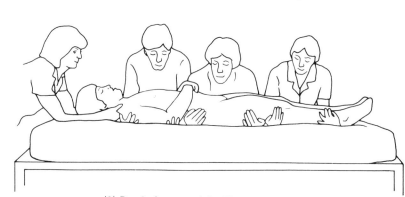

(3) Ready for a straight lift.

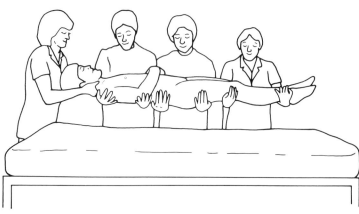

(4) Straight lift.

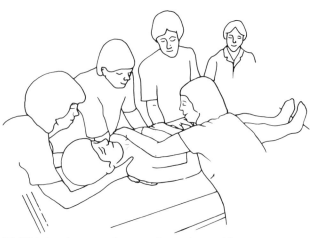

(5) Withdrawing arms from under patient, with counter traction to prevent movement of spine.

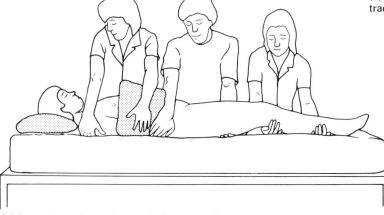

(6) Preparing to log roll paraplegic patient. For tetraplegic patient, head hold is also needed.

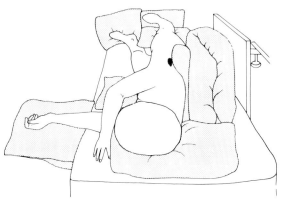

(7) Completed log roll, patient in lateral position.

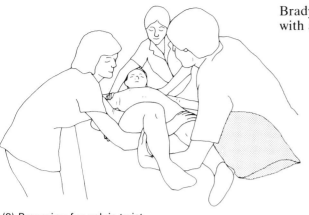

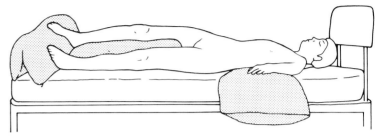

(8) Preparing for pelvic twist.

(9) Pelvic twist completed.

Bradycardia may be exacerbated when turning a newly injured patient with a high lesion on to the left side.

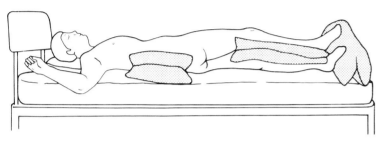

(10) Pelvic twist completed: side view of patient showing folded pillows to maintain position—sacrum free of pressure.

Note: In all lifts and turns the person holding the head is in charge of the timing and coordination of the team. The frequency of turns is determined by the patient's tolerance, usually two to three hours initially, but with increasing intervals as long as no marking occurs. By the time the patient is discharged it is hoped that turning at night will not be needed.

The pelvic twist is a simple turn, needing only three nurses to perform, and suitable for many tetraplegic patients. It must not be used in thoracolumbar lesions. The nurse at the patient's head holds the shoulders securely on to the bed; the second nurse applies counter pressure and gets ready to support the back and legs on completion of the twist before inserting the pillows. The third nurse proceeds with the twist by placing her or his upper arm under the patient's back (using counter pressure) and her or his lower arm under the patient's nearest thigh and over the furthest to support the hip (8). The movement is a gentle lift and turn of the near hip joint, enough to free the sacrum of any pressure. On completion of the turn two pillows are placed under the upper leg and one folded into the lumbar region to support the pelvis (9 and 10).

Care of the limbs

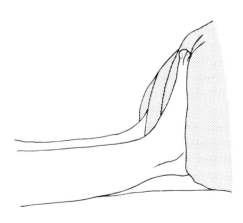

Heel is free of pressure with the foot held at 90°.

Legs

When patients are supine: (a) avoid hyperextension of the knees; (b) keep the feet in line with the hips; and (c) hold the foot at 90° using foot boards and pillows, avoiding pressure on the heels.

When patients are on their side: (a) the lower leg should be extended and (b) the upper leg should be slightly flexed, lying on a pillow and not over the lower leg.

Arms

When tetraplegic patients are supine the joints need to be placed in a full range of positions and the hands and arms must always be supported.

When patients are lying on their side both arms should be positioned forward and supported on pillows. The underlying shoulder is protected from pressure by being pulled gently forward or by an axillary pillow, or both.

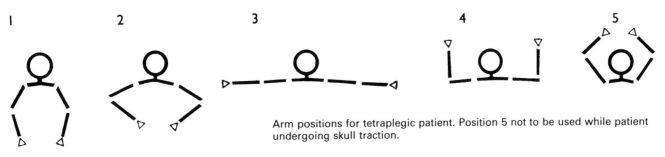

Arm positions for tetraplegic patient. Position 5 not to be used while patient undergoing skull traction.

General educational and preventive measures

Skin and pressure
- Examine and relieve pressure regularly
- Keep clean
- Avoid damage
- Treat minor abrasions/injuries

Sensory deprivation
- Familiarisation with surroundings/ interpretation of incoming stimuli
- Highest cognitive functioning
- Reality orientation
- Active role in care

Nutrition
- Encourage and help patient to eat high protein diet
- Involve dietitian for further help
- Enteral feeding if necessary
- Nutritional education—feeding aids
                                    —diet

Bladder management
- Asepsis to prevent infection
- Achieve fluid balance (intake and output according to catheter)

Indwelling urethral catheter ⎱ aim—output at
Suprapubic catheter   ⎰ least 3 1/day

Intermittent catheterisation—aim—output no more than 500 ml at each catheterisation, to prevent overdistension

---

Skin and pressure

Skin cleanliness is fundamental and good long term arrangements for bathing or showering must be made. "Minor" skin infections should be treated and fingernails and toenails cared for—ingrowing toenails are particularly common. Patients must be taught about the hazards of sensory loss and the need to inspect their skin and extremities regularly. They must be taught to be conscious of pressure, and must understand that the risk of pressure sores increases during periods of physical or emotional distress, depression, tiredness, and intercurrent illnesses.

Education is also important to enable the patient to select suitable clothing, with sore prevention and poikilothermia in mind.

Internal environment

Patients with high thoracic and cervical lesions remain susceptible to respiratory complications, and a health education programme should be implemented with the long term goal of reducing the risk of chest infections.

Nursing care also involves monitoring the patient for evidence of deep vein thrombosis. This includes observing and measuring the calves and thighs, but in paraplegia a raised temperature is sometimes the only indication that thromboembolic complications may be developing.

Profound loss of sensation below the level of the lesion, a restricted visual field due to the enforced bed rest, unfamiliar surroundings, and many interruptions imposed on newly injured patients in the early stages may cause sensory deprivation leading to confusion and disorientation.

The aim is to try and redress the balance by increasing the sensory input to the patient. Many tools can be used, one of them being that of touch, in a caring comforting manner, above the level of the lesion. Mirrors can be placed strategically to extend the field of vision, and reality training employed, using clocks, calendars, newspapers, the involvement of friends and relatives and, most important, allowing the patient to have a decision making role.

Nutrition

Life threatening conditions in the initial acute phase often overshadow the nutritional needs of the patient. The risk factors associated with trauma, the initial period of paralytic ileus, anorexia, and the inability to use the hands in high lesions can all lead to malnutrition and severe weight loss. The nursing goal in the acute phase is to maintain nutritional support by: (a) encouraging and helping to feed the patient with a high protein diet; (b) involving the dietician if further nutritional assistance is required; and (c) implementing enteral feeding when necessary. In the rehabilitation phase the nurse needs to be familiar with feeding aids provided by the occupational therapist and to implement an individual nutritional education programme.

Bladder management

The management of the bladder is concerned, firstly, with preventing urinary tract infection. This is an extreme challenge in the neuropathic bladder, and a strict aseptic technique is vital. Careful handwashing between patients, the use of gloves when emptying drainage bags, and the use of a closed drainage system are all part of good practice. Perineal toilet using soap and water, particularly after bowel evacuation, will reduce pathogenic skin flora.

Care of the bladder includes performing catheterisations. This technique can be performed by nurses, but a specific training programme is required. Care also includes managing the fluid balance appropriate to the individual—for example, fluid restriction during intermittent catheterisation to prevent overdistension of the bladder, or high fluid intake for patients with indwelling catheters to minimise the dangers of infection and calculus formation. Finally, nurses can help in educating patients to understand their bladders, to recognise when something is wrong, and to teach them how to order and care for their appliances.

Achieving continence in women presents a greater problem than in men, particularly for some females in the premenstrual phase and during menstruation. Self intermittent catheterisation is the best method if this is possible and practicable, but careful control of fluids and a daily routine will be needed to maintain dryness between catheterisations. Suprapubic catheters are sometimes considered for sexual and aesthetic reasons and to prevent urethral damage.

Bowel care

During the period of spinal shock the bowel is flaccid, so it must not be allowed to overdistend causing constipation with overflow incontinence. An initial rectal check is made to ascertain whether faeces are present; if they are they should be manually evacuated. Manual bowel evacuation thereafter will continue daily or on alternate days during the period in bed. Very little bowel activity will be expected for the first two or three days. Evacuation should be performed using plenty of lubricant and with only one gloved finger inserted into the anus. Trauma, including anal fissure formation and a split natal cleft, is possible if insufficient care is taken. Suppositories to lubricate the faeces and aperients may be required to achieve an evacuation. The training programme depends on whether the bowel empties reflexly or is flaccid, and on what level of self care the patient is likely to achieve.

Sexuality

After a spinal cord lesion patients need to redefine sexuality and all that it encompasses. Nurses have to recognise when patients are ready to discuss sexuality and respond appropriately. This need is not always verbalised in the early stages and often manifests itself only in sexual innuendo. Discussion should be encouraged and should include dispelling myths, exploring the patient's "new" sexual status, identifying problems, and advising on how to deal with them. Referral to medical staff and other agencies for further information and management should be made as appropriate.

Bowel

Upper motor neurone lesion

Reflex emptying—after suppositories or digital stimulation

May not need aperients if diet appropriate

Lower motor neurone lesion

Flaccid

Manual evacuation and aperients usually required but may be able to empty, using abdominal muscles

Suppositories ineffective

Sexuality

- Redefine sexuality
- Dispel myths
- Educate
- Promote/employ alternatives

PHYSIOTHERAPY

Trudy Ward, David Grundy

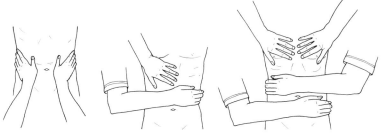

Assisted coughing—Careful coordination and communication between physiotherapist and patient is vital if these techniques are to be successful. (1) The therapist's hands are placed just below the ribs and, as the patient attempts to cough, the therapist pushes inwards and upwards to reinforce the patient's cough. Care must be taken not to press down on to the abdomen. (2) The hands are placed either side of the lower ribs, and the forearm used to push inwards and upwards as the patient coughs. (3) Two people may be needed to treat the patient with tenacious sputum, or a wide chest wall. The therapists should be positioned on either side of the patient, each with one arm below the ribs, and the other on the upper chest wall.

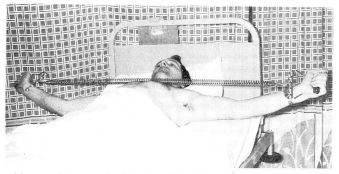

Patient with complete paraplegia below T5 pulling chest expander. Bilateral arm strengthening exercises must be done in supine position to maintain vertebral alignment.

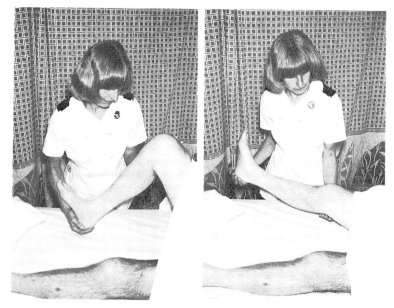

Passive movements to a patient's leg. Good support must be given to the paralysed joints and a full range of movement achieved.

Physiotherapy assessment and treatment should be carried out as soon as possible after injury. During the early acute stage, care of the chest and paralysed limbs is of prime importance. Chest complications may occur as a result of the accident—for example, from inhaling water during diving incidents, from local complications such as fractured ribs, or from respiratory insufficiency caused by the level of the injury. Pre-existing lung disease may further complicate respiration.

All patients receive prophylactic chest treatment, which includes deep breathing exercises, percussion, and coughing, assisted if necessary. Careful monitoring is essential for tetraplegic patients as cord oedema may result in an ascending level of paralysis, further compromising respiration.

Patients with tetraplegia or high level paraplegia may have paralysed abdominal and intercostal muscles and will be unable to cough effectively. Assisted coughing will be necessary for effective lung clearance.

All paralysed limbs are moved passively each day to maintain a full range of movement. Loss of sensation means that joints and soft tissues are vulnerable to overstretching, so great care must be taken not to cause trauma.

Provided that stability of the bony injury is maintained, passive hip stretching with the patient in the lateral position, and strengthening of non-paralysed muscle groups, is encouraged.

An appropriate wheelchair is ordered during the stage of bed rest. This stage is of great value in establishing rapport with the patient, which is necessary for efficient rehabilitation and will not be achieved unless the patient has complete confidence in his or her therapist.

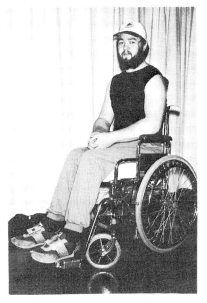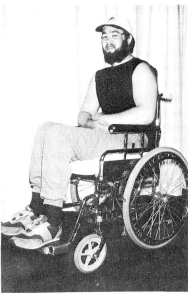

Left: Patient correctly seated in wheelchair—erect and well back in the chair; footplates are level and adjusted to allow thighs to be fully supported on wheelchair cushion and for weight to be evenly distributed. Heel loops prevent the feet falling backwards off the footplates. Right: Patient seated incorrectly—"slumped" and with poor trunk posture. Footplates are too high so there is excessive pressure on the sacrum—a potential pressure problem.

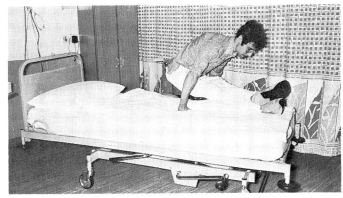

Patient with complete paraplegia below T12 transferring on to the bed. Having first lifted legs up on to the bed the patient then lifts rest of body horizontally from chair to bed. Hand position is important to achieve a safe lift, avoiding contact with wheel.

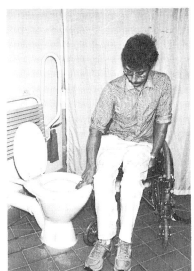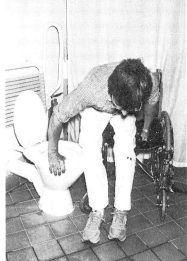

Patient with complete paraplegia below T12 transferring on to the toilet. Toilet seat must be well padded. Chair and legs must be carefully positioned to ensure a safe lift. Patient has to lift and rotate in one movement, so balance must be good and shoulder strength maximal.

Once the bony injury is stable patients will start sitting, preferably using a profiling bed, before getting up into a wheelchair. This is a gradual process because of the possibility of postural hypotension, which is most severe in patients with an injury above T6 and in the elderly.

Once a patient is in a wheelchair regular relief of pressure at the ischial, trochanteric, and sacral regions is essential to prevent the development of pressure sores in the absence of sensation. Patients must be taught to lift themselves to relieve pressure every 15 minutes. This must become a permanent habit. Paraplegic patients can usually do this without help by lifting on the wheels or arm rests of their wheelchairs. Tetraplegic patients should initially be provided with a cushion giving adequate pressure relief, but may in time be able to relieve pressure themselves.

Physical rehabilitation includes the following:

(1) Familiarity with the wheelchair. The patient has to be taught how to propel the chair, operate the brakes, remove the footplates and armrests, and fold and transport the wheelchair. Basic skills include pushing on level and sloping ground and turning the chair.

(2) Relearning the ability to balance. The length of time this takes will depend on the degree of loss of proprioception and on trunk control.

(3) Strengthening non-paralysed muscles.

(4) Learning to transfer from wheelchair to bed, toilet, bath, floor, easy chair, and car. Teaching these skills is only possible once confidence in balance is achieved and there is sufficient strength in the arms and shoulder girdles. The degree of independence achieved by each patient will depend on factors such as the level of the lesion, the degree of spasticity, body size and weight, age, mental attitude, and the skill of the therapist. Patients who cannot transfer themselves will require help, and patient and helpers will spend time with therapists and nurses learning the techniques for pressure relief, dressing, transferring, and various wheelchair manoeuvres. The level of independence achievable by tetraplegic patients is charted on page 41. Close cooperation between physiotherapists and occupational therapists helps patients to reach their full potential.

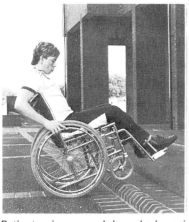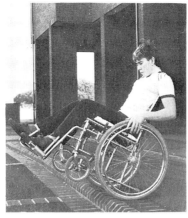

Patient going up and down kerb unaided—must be able to balance on the rear wheels and travel forwards while maintaining this position and then have enough strength to push chair up kerb and lower it down in controlled manner.

(5) Learning advanced wheelchair skills: (a) backwheel balancing to allow easier manoeuvrability over rough ground and provide a means of negotiating kerbs; (b) jumping the chair sideways for manoeuvrability in a limited space; and (c) lifting the wheelchair in and out of a car unaided.

(6) Regular standing, which helps to prevent contractures, reduce spasticity, and minimise osteoporosis. In patients subject to postural hypotension the vertical position must be assumed gradually, and patients may be helped by the use of an abdominal binder. The tilt table is used initially, patients progressing to an Oswestry standing frame later.

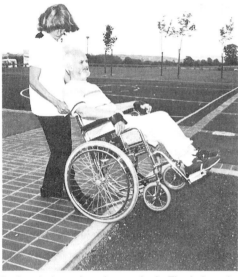

Patient being taken down a kerb. The helper tips the chair back on to its rear wheels and lowers it down the kerb, keeping the chair balanced throughout.

Patients with low thoracic or lumbar lesions may be suitable for gait training using calipers and crutches, but success will depend on the patient's age, height, weight, degree of spasticity, and attitude. Orthotic devices such as the reciprocating gait orthosis (RGO) and hip guidance orthosis (HGO) may be considered for patients including those unsuitable for traditional calipers and crutches. Checks should be made on all patients and their orthoses at regular intervals.

Wheelchair design has been much influenced by technology. Lightweight wheelchairs are more aesthetically acceptable, considerably easier to use, and often adjustable to the individual user's requirements.

Sporting activities can be a valuable part of rehabilitation as they encourage balance, strength, and fitness, plus a sense of camaraderie and may well help patients reintegrate into society once they leave hospital. Archery, darts, snooker, table tennis, fencing, swimming, wheelchair basketball, and other athletic pursuits are all possible and are encouraged.

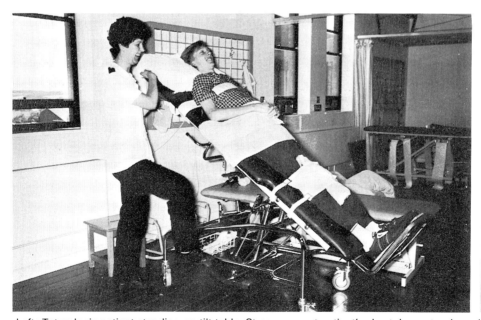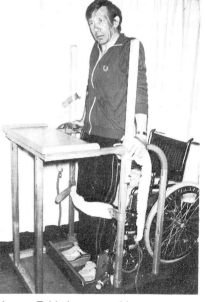

Left: Tetraplegic patient standing on tilt table. Straps support patient's chest, lower trunk, and knees. Table is operated by therapist, the fully upright position being achieved gradually. Right: Oswestry standing frame enables paraplegic patient to stand by providing support through suitably placed padded straps at toes and heels, knees, and gluteal region. Uprights and two further straps allow a tetraplegic patient to stand in the frame by supporting the trunk.

Special problems

Incomplete lesions

Patients with incomplete lesions are a great challenge to physiotherapists as they present in various ways, which necessitates individual planning of treatment and continuing assessment. Patients with incomplete lesions may remain severely disabled despite neurological recovery. Spasticity may restrict the functional use of limbs despite apparently good isolated muscle power. The absence of proprioception or sensory appreciation will also hinder functional ability in the presence of otherwise adequate muscle power. Patients with a central cord lesion may be able to walk, but weakness in the arms may prevent them from dressing, feeding, or protecting themselves from falls. Recovery may well continue over several months, if not years, so careful review and referral to the patient's district physiotherapy department may be necessary to enable full functional potential to be achieved.

Children

Spinal cord injury in children is rare. The most important principles in the physical rehabilitation of the growing child with a spinal cord injury are preventing deformities, particularly scoliosis, and encouraging growth of the long bones. To achieve these aims the child requires careful bracing and full length calipers to maintain an upright posture for as much of the day as possible. The child should be provided with a means of walking such as: (a) brace and calipers with crutches or rollator, (b) a swivel walker, or (c) hip guidance orthosis or reciprocating gait orthosis.

Sitting should be discouraged to prevent vertebral deformity. A wheelchair should be provided, however, to facilitate social activity both in and out of the home. Return to normal schooling is encouraged as soon as possible.

Young children have arms that are relatively short in relation to the trunk, so they should not attempt independent transfers. The child may therefore need to be readmitted and taught transfer skills at a later stage. Continued follow up is necessary throughout childhood, adolescence, and early adult life to ensure that adjustments are made to braces, calipers, and wheelchair to maintain good posture and correct growth.

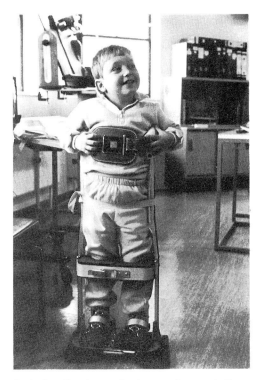

Swivel walker leaves both arms free and allows the child to travel over flat ground by rotating the shoulders alternately.

Gait expectations of patients with complete paraplegia

All patients should be totally independent with all transfers and chair manoeuvres both indoors and outdoors.

Level of injury	Gait used	Descriptions
T1-T8	Gait—swing to with calipers and rollator May use crutches if spasticity is controlled	*Swing to gait* is the easiest type of gait to achieve but is slow and used only as an exercise. The patient puts the crutches a short distance in front of the feet and leans forward on to the crutches. He or she then pushes down with the shoulders, which lifts both legs together. The feet must land behind the crutches. It is a short, sharp lift. Prolonging the lift will make the feet go past the crutches and the patient will lose balance and fall.
T8-T10	Swing to and swing through gait with full length calipers and crutches Walking more likely to be an exercise rather than fully functional	*Swing through gait* is for speed and is the most functional for walking outside. However, it does expend a lot of energy. The patient places the crutches about 18 inches in front of the feet and leans forward on to the crutches; he or she then pushes the shoulder down, which raises both feet off the floor together. The lift must be maintained so that the feet are placed the same distance in front of the crutches as they started behind. As the feet touch the floor the patient must retract the shoulders to extend the hips and hence remain balanced.
T10-L2	Swing through and four point with calipers and crutches Requires wheelchair for part of day—walking may be fully functional	
L2-L4	Below knee calipers with crutches or sticks Wheelchair not required	*Four point gait* is the most difficult and requires excellent balance and strong shoulders and trunk. It is the nearest equivalent to a normal gait, but is very slow. The patient moves one crutch forward, transfers body weight on to the adjacent leg, and then moves the opposite leg forward by using latissimus dorsi to "hitch" the hip. The step must be short; if too large a step is taken the patient will fall, as he or she cannot recover balance.
L4-L5	May or may not require calipers Wheelchair not required May require sticks or other walking aid	

All the above depend on age, stature, amount and control of spasticity, any pre-existing medical condition and the individual's motivation.

OCCUPATIONAL THERAPY

Jane Henshaw, David Grundy

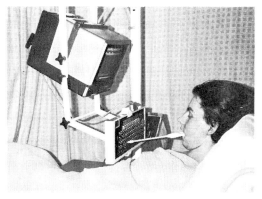

An overbed computer and word processor can be used by patients with any level of injury.

The months after a severe spinal cord injury are invariably an extremely difficult period for patients as they gradually adjust to what will probably be a lifetime of disability.

Occupational therapists are particularly concerned with helping patients reach the highest levels of physical and psychological independence that their injuries, homes, and work environments will allow. The degree of involvement will depend largely on the neurological level of the spinal lesion, but the occupational therapist's skill is particularly important in managing tetraplegic patients, in whom limited function in the arms can seriously hamper the common activities of daily living such as washing, dressing, and feeding. However, by the use of various aids and adaptations to the home and place of work some of these difficulties can be overcome successfully.

The paraplegic patient obviously requires less of the occupational therapist's time, the main concerns being home modifications, return to work, driving, and introducing sport and leisure activities. None of these aims can be achieved in isolation and therefore close working relationships with physiotherapists are essential.

Splinting

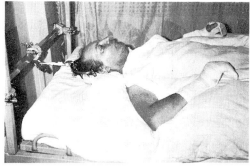

Tetraplegic hands are splinted as soon as possible, this continuing throughout the period of rehabilitation.

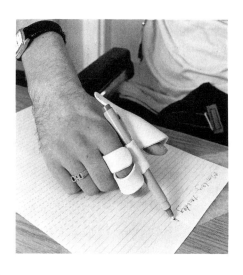

Splints are essential for tetraplegic patients to maintain their hands in the optimum position for function. Splints are made as soon as possible after a patient's admission to the spinal injuries unit and are worn during the period of bed rest, for increasing periods of time depending on the patient's tolerance. Once patients are mobilised into wheelchairs they should still wear the splints at night, as even at this stage irreversible flexion contractures of the metacarpophalangeal and interphalangeal joints may occur.

Many tetraplegic patients also need a variety of splints, such as writing or typing splints and wrist support splints, feeding straps, and pushing gloves, to enable them to carry out normal daily activities. All splints are made individually for each patient by the therapist.

Patient with complete tetraplegia below C6, using individually designed writing splint.

Home visit and home alterations

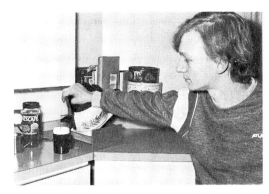

Simple tipping device enables tetraplegic patient to use a kettle safely.

Contact with the community physician and local social services department before a visit to the patient's home to assess its suitability for both short and long term wheelchair occupation is advisable as soon as possible after injury. This initial visit should involve a team from the spinal injuries unit, consisting of the occupational therapist and the social worker, and also representatives from the patient's home area—the local domiciliary occupational therapist and social worker, as well as the patient's family. It is far from ideal that the patient is not included on this visit, but if there is to be any reasonable chance of the alterations being completed before the patient's discharge from hospital (usually four to nine months) the visit needs to take place well before the patient is fit to travel to his or her home. Nevertheless, no final recommendations should be made until all aspects have been fully discussed with the patient.

Depending on the family's financial circumstances, grant aid towards the alterations may be available from the patient's local council or social services department. Once the decision has been made about the adaptations required, plans need to be drawn up so that alterations can start as early as possible.

Wheelchairs and cushions

Types of wheelchair

Department of Health approved manual, eg Carters	Supplied by the health authority through local district wheelchair service
Manual lightweight	About half the weight of the approved chair; easier to propel and adjust; better looking; requires private funding
Electrically operated for functional mobility in high tetraplegia (C5 and above)	Model for home or institutional use supplied by the wheelchair service
	Model for outdoor use requires private funding

During the initial period of bed rest the patient is assessed for a wheelchair. The patient's weight, height, and expected functional ability are taken into account when deciding on the type of chair required. If an electric wheelchair might also be necessary application for this is delayed until later in the patient's rehabilitation, when his or her needs can be evaluated more accurately. A stock of electrically and manually operated wheelchairs should be held in the spinal injuries unit for assessment purposes.

Although a 10 cm foam or pincore latex cushion is normally ordered with the wheelchair, it is not always satisfactory because of unacceptable interface pressures under the ischial tuberosities, and it may need to be changed to a more suitable type such as a Jay or Roho cushion. A wide range of cushions should be stocked in the unit to meet all requirements, so that the appropriate one may be obtained for the patient. It is emphasised to the patient that the cushion should be reviewed regularly.

Activities of daily living

Functional ability and expected level of independence of tetraplegic patients

Level of injury

Complete lesion below C3	Totally dependent Diaphragm paralysed, needs tracheostomy with permanent ventilation or diaphragm pacing Chin or breath controlled electric wheelchair required
Complete lesion below C4	Totally dependent Can breathe independently using diaphragm Can shrug shoulders Can use electric wheelchair with chin control Can type/use computer using a mouth stick Needs environmental control system (such as Possum) to turn on lights, open doors, etc operated by shoulder shrug or mouthpiece
Complete lesion below C5	Can move shoulders and flex elbows Can feed with a feeding strap/universal cuff Can wash face, comb hair, clean teeth—using feeding strap/universal cuff Can write using individually designed splint and wrist support Can help in dressing upper half of body Can push manual wheelchair short distances on the flat, provided that pushing gloves are used with capstan rims on the wheels May be able to transfer across level surfaces, using sliding board and a helper Electric wheelchair needed for functional mobility

Level of injury

Complete lesion below C6	Can extend wrists Still needs strap to feed and for self care Can write using individually designed splint, but may not need wrist support Can dress upper half of body unaided Can help in dressing lower half of body Can propel wheelchair up gentle slopes Can be independent in bed, car, and toilet transfers Can drive with hand controls
Complete lesion below C7	Full wrist movement and some hand function, but no finger flexion or fine hand movements Can do all transfers, feed, and dress independently Can drive with hand controls
Complete lesion below C8	All hand muscles except intrinsics preserved Wheelchair independent, but difficulty in going up and down kerbs Can drive with hand controls
Complete lesion below T1	Complete innervation of arms Totally independent wheelchair life Can drive with hand controls

These expectations are general and depend on the patient's age, sex, physical proportions, physical condition before injury, degree of spasticity, and motivation.

Occupational therapy

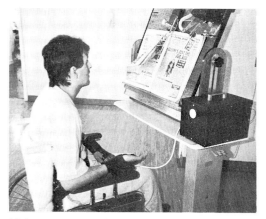

Light pressure on the control switch (under the right forearm) activates the page turner.

Once patients are out of bed and physically strong all but those with the highest lesions are taught to dress. When possible tetraplegic patients are taught to feed, drink, wash, brush their hair, clean their teeth, and shave. They are also taught to sign their names, type, and use a computer, the telephone, and when necessary page turners and other forms of environmental control.

Very high lesions

Patients with very high lesions are now surviving, some requiring domiciliary ventilation. They present a tremendous challenge to occupational therapists, who must endeavour to teach them to be as independent as possible with the aid of mouth sticks and breath control. Modern computer technology has enabled this group of patients to enjoy a far better quality of life.

Recreation

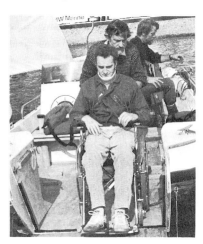

Leisure activities are if anything more important for disabled than for ablebodied people. Many patients with spinal cord injuries are unemployed and therefore have more leisure time available. To maintain their self esteem suitable hobbies and sporting activities should be encouraged. Activities that patients might have considered impossible may be pursued with a little thought and suitable adjustment—for example, a camera with an automatic winding device, tripod lead, and bracket to attach the camera to the wheelchair can enable a tetraplegic patient to have an interest in photography. Leisure pursuits involving patients with spinal cord injuries and ablebodied people should also be encouraged to maintain the competitive instinct and to help integration back into the community.

Work

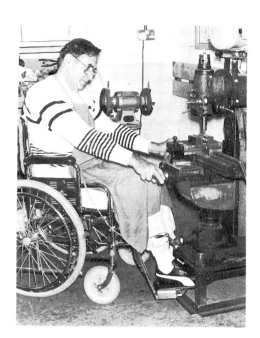

Paraplegic patient working milling machine.

Work is of varying importance to patients, but most will see it as giving a sense of purpose to their life and will want to return to their former occupation if at all possible. Early contact with the patient's employer to discuss the feasibility of eventual return to his or her previous job is important. If the degree of a patient's disability precludes this, some employers are sympathetic and flexible and will offer a job that will be possible from a wheelchair. However, many patients find life outside hospital difficult enough initially, without the added responsibility of a job, and in these circumstances a period of adjustment at home is advisable before they return to work, as it may be two or three years or longer before a patient is psychologically rehabilitated.

When such patients feel ready to consider some alternative employment they can contact their local disability employment adviser. If a patient is planning to return to his or her previous employer, school, or college the occupational therapist should assess the suitability of the premises for wheelchair accessibility. Recommendations are then made to the placement, assessment, and counselling team (PACT) or local education authority if alterations to the buildings or the installation of specialised equipment are needed to make them suitable for the patient.

Ideally, if patients are considering returning to work they should spend some time in a rehabilitation workshop. In this environment they should be able to test their aptitude for activities such as carpentry, engineering, and electronics and for using computers, word processors, and other products of modern technology. In addition, patients will build up their strength and stamina and both they and the staff will have a clearer idea of their employment capabilities.

SOCIAL NEEDS OF PATIENT AND FAMILY

Erica Bamford, David Grundy

The aim of successful rehabilitation is to enable the patient to live as satisfactory and fulfilling a life as possible. This will mean different choices and decisions for each individual depending on the degree of disability, the family and social environment, and preferred lifestyle.

The vast majority of patients want to live in their own homes and not in residential care, and very severely disabled people achieve this successfully. Many will live as part of a family, or increasingly choose to live independently with support from community services. *Caring for People* (Cm 849, 1989) recognises this, and since 1988 the Independent Living Fund has made payments to people with severe disabilities to enable them to purchase care to supplement that provided by family and local health and social services. The Independent Living Fund will end on 31 March 1993, and it has been said in parliament that a new organisation will be established to make payments to current recipients only. The position for new applicants is uncertain.

Where patients are living	%
Living with relatives after discharge	69
Living independently after discharge	21
Chose long term residential care after discharge	0
Required interim residential care on discharge	17
Still in interim care	5
Transferred to other hospital	5

Some patients appear in more than one category. Figures derived from new injury discharges from Duke of Cornwall Spinal Treatment Centre 1990-1.

For most people spinal cord injury demands changes in almost every aspect of life—personal relationships, the physical structure of the home, work and education, social and leisure pursuits, and financial management. Consequently, exhaustive and careful planning by the spinal unit staff and staff responsible for community services, in conjunction with the patient and family, is essential. Because of the complexities and scale of what is required, this planning should start as soon after injury as possible. Planning before discharge is only the start of a lifelong, probably fluctuating, need for services. In providing these the social and emotional wellbeing of the person and family must be considered along with physical health. Physical health supports and is supported by a satisfactory lifestyle.

Changed relationships

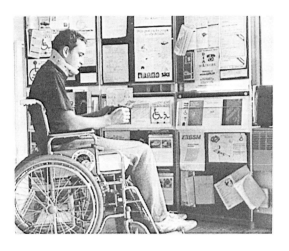

The onset of severe disability can have profound effects, not necessarily damaging, on existing personal relationships and on the formation of new relationships. Disability will change the roles people have in a relationship: for instance, a wife whose husband is disabled may find that she has to manage the family's financial and business affairs for the first time, or a husband whose wife has been injured may have to undertake extra household tasks. The ablebodied person—husband, wife, or parent—may have to provide intimate personal care. The workload of everyone concerned is likely to be much greater. For many couples an active and satisfying sexual relationship will be possible, but it will be different. These changes, in addition to the feelings engendered by loss of function and its actual cause, are likely to have major repercussions.

Many spinal cord injuries happen to late adolescents or young adults at the stage when they are beginning to form relationships with the opposite sex and establish independence from parents, and when they may be very concerned about their ability to do so. It takes time and the realisation that people do think that they are still worthwhile before necessary self esteem can return. These adjustments are likely to take place after discharge from hospital, because then the issues become clearer. Many people find that the initial period after discharge can be very stressful.

Social needs

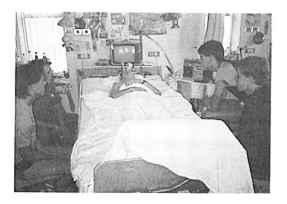

Good community support, including practical help with the tasks of caring, and also the imaginative provision of resources to enable the person and carers to participate in normal community activities, are likely to help the process. Tired people who have limited social satisfactions will find it more difficult to make the necessary adjustments. Counselling can be a valuable source of help in making these adjustments. Studies indicate that people with spinal cord injuries are not as psychologically distressed or depressed by their injury as ablebodied people, including experienced staff, think them to be.

It is important to remember that many people with spinal cord injury do lead active fulfilling lives, though this may take time to achieve.

Finance

Benefits commonly available to disabled people

Benefits to assist with disability

Disability living allowance (DS 704)
Attendance allowance (if over 65 years of age) (DS 702)
Disability working allowance (DS 703)

Industrial disablement benefit (FB 15; NI 6)
Help with NHS charges and free prescriptions and travel to hospital (AG 1, A 11, and H 11)

Income maintenance benefits
(1) *a* Statutory sick pay (for 28 weeks) (NI 244) if in employment and not self employed
 or
 Sickness benefit (for 28 weeks) (NI 16) if self employed or unemployed } Depending on sufficient national insurance
 b Invalidity benefit (NI 16A) (after 28 weeks) } contributions

(2) If not enough contributions:
 Income support (28 weeks) (IS 1) means tested
 Severe disablement allowance (if eligible) (NI 252)
 Income support will "top up" any of the above if income is below the assessed needs level

(3) War disablement pension (FB 16) and (MPL 153)

(4) Housing benefit and community charge benefit (administered by district councils) (CCB 1)

(5) Invalid care allowance (DS 700) (paid to some carers)

(6) Family credit (FC 1) If working, on low income, and with dependent children.

(DSS leaflet numbers are given in parentheses)

Adequate finance is a major factor in determining successful rehabilitation, but many severely disabled people are living in poverty.

Not only do patients and their families have to cope with all the stresses of injury; they may also have to live on a severely reduced income which cannot support their existing lifestyle. In addition, it is more expensive to live as a disabled person. Disability living allowance, or attendance allowance for over 65 year olds, provides some help with the more obvious costs, but no provision exists for tasks such as household decorating, simple repairs, and gardening, which the disabled person may no longer be able to do.

Even if the person receives financial compensation, this will take several years to be granted, and though interim payments can be made in some circumstances they are not always available at the time of discharge from hospital, when there is likely to be major expenditure on either moving or adapting the present house.

Because of the interruption in, or possible loss of, earning capacity many people will be dependent for long periods on welfare benefits administered by the Department of Social Security. These are complex, and various studies have shown that many disabled people are receiving less than their entitlement, sometimes by quite substantial amounts. It is therefore important for those working with disabled people to be aware that they may be underclaiming benefits and to advise them accordingly.

Adapting homes

	%
Able to return to own home with adaptations	46
Had to move to live with relatives	8
Required rehousing, provided by district council	27
Required rehousing, patient or family bought property	9
Required rehousing, provided by housing associations or through private renting	10

Figures derived from new injury discharges from Duke of Cornwall Spinal Treatment Centre 1990-1.

Most houses are unsuitable for wheelchairs unless adapted. This presents a continuing problem because, though patients may return to an adapted house or be rehoused from hospital, they may well want to change house in the future, especially as spinal cord injuries typically occur in young people, who would normally move house several times. A disabled person may have considerable difficulty in finding a suitable house, and there can be time restrictions on further provision of grants for adaptations. Many cannot afford to buy a house and will depend on council housing, housing association property, or privately rented property, all of which are in short supply. Consequently, any move of house can be difficult to achieve and has to be planned well ahead. The services of community occupational therapists, housing departments, and social workers may be required.

Employment

	%
In work	31
Returned to work, now unemployed	4
In education or training	22
Voluntary work	11
No employment	32

Figures based on survey by Rosemarie Castle, Dip COT, of patients discharged from Duke of Cornwall Spinal Treatment Centre (1991).

Information and advice on benefits

Department of Social Security
 (local office or DSS benefit enquiry line
 0800 882 200)
Citizens Advice Bureaux
Social services departments of local councils
Disablement Income Group (DIG)
 Millmead Business Centre, Millmead Road,
 London N17 9QU (081 801 8013)
DIG (Scotland), ECAS House,
 28-30 Howden Street
 Edinburgh EH8 9HW (031 667 0249)
DIAL (disabled information and advice line)
 [Name of town]. A voluntary organisation
 operating in some areas.

Disability Rights Handbook (Price £6.95, post free.)
 Published annually by the Disability Alliance
 Educational and Research Association,
 Universal House, 88-94 Wentworth Street,
 London E1 7SA (071 247 8776)
Spinal Injuries Association, Newpoint House,
 76 St James's Lane, London N10 3DF
 (081 444 2121)
Other local voluntary advice centres, many
 listed in *Disability Rights Handbook*.

Employment is possible for severely disabled people, and for some the sense of achievement and satisfaction gained from work is crucial to their self esteem. For others work is unimportant and coping with disability is challenging enough. A minority are able and keen to return to the work they were doing before the injury. It is important not to underestimate the adjustments of returning to live in the community and not to start work too quickly. The placement, assessment, and counselling teams (PACTs) and disablement employment advisers (DEAs) of the Employment Service provide advice and financial help to employers to make necessary adaptations to the place of work to enable the person to resume employment.

Many people will have to establish new careers, or will not yet have started work. It can take considerable time, up to two or three years, to make sufficient physical and psychological adjustment to undertake an entirely new training or career. The careers service or Employment Service, including the services mentioned above, can provide careers guidance and help in finding employment. People with disabilities find it much more difficult to find work, and a high proportion of those wanting to work are unemployed.

A considerable number of statutory services are concerned with providing services for disabled people. Voluntary organisations also provide important resources. They can act as pressure and self help groups, and organisations of disabled people have the knowledge and understanding born of personal experience. There are many such organisations, of which the Spinal Injuries Association is particularly relevant.

To mobilise and coordinate these services, which often vary in what they can provide in different geographical areas, is a major undertaking. Too often disabled people fail to receive a service that would be of benefit or they may feel overwhelmed and not in control of their own lives, with consequent damage to morale and health. Disabled people and their families should have access to full information about the services available and be enabled to make their own decisions about what they need.

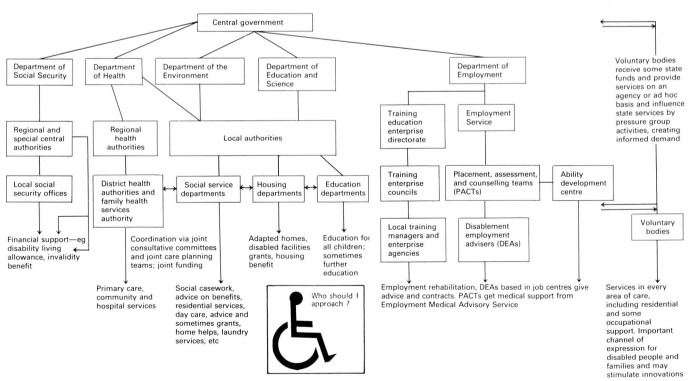

Adapted from Office of Health Economics. *Mental Handicap: Ways Forward*. 1978.

TRANSFER OF CARE FROM HOSPITAL TO COMMUNITY

Hilary Dover, David Grundy

Discharge from hospital is a complicated process for both paraplegic and tetraplegic patients. Physical care is a major concern, and here the difference between levels of injury is profound. Paraplegic people usually become self caring; those with low tetraplegia, especially if young, may also achieve independence, but those with high tetraplegia need someone else to take care of their physical needs to varying degrees.

Achieving good care depends largely on educating the patients, their families, and the community staff. Patients should be expert at understanding and, as far as possible, caring for their own bodies. They need to be able to recognise potential problems and either deal with them themselves or know where to go for advice.

Much time is spent in teaching the importance of good skin, bladder, and bowel care, as long term problems in these areas are common.

People need to develop skills in:

- Understanding and caring for their own bodies
- Recognising potential problems
- Dealing with problems or learning where to go for advice

Patient education

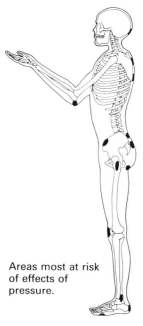

Areas most at risk of effects of pressure.

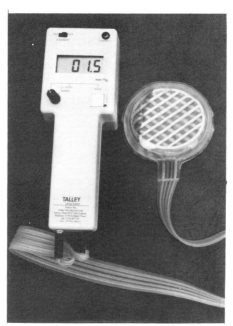

Above right: Talley skin pressure evaluator to measure pressure between the skin and supporting surface. Right: Talley skin pressure evaluator about to be positioned under the patient's ischial tuberosity; 60 mm Hg is safe for patients who can lift themselves to relieve pressure and 35 mm Hg for those who cannot, the choice of cushion being decided in part by these measurements.

Skin care

Patients are taught how to use a mirror to check the pressure areas regularly. Wheelchairs and cushions are best assessed in a pressure clinic. If patients cannot lift themselves in their chair they need a cushion that allows them to sit in their wheelchair all day without producing a red mark on the skin. Weight, muscle size, activity, ability to lift in the wheelchair, nutrition, and posture all affect the type of cushion needed.

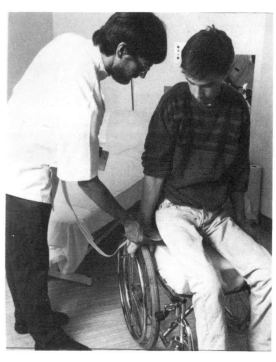

Clothes should be made of natural fibre because many patients sweat excessively; and trousers must not be tight, otherwise there is a risk of pressure sores in the groin or elsewhere from tight seams. Shoes should generally be one size larger than before the injury, otherwise pressure marks on the feet are liable to occur. The choice of a suitable mattress is also very important. Many pressure spreading mattresses are now available, so all patients should be able to sleep for at least six hours without being turned. Advice from the pressure clinic remains available to patients at every outpatient appointment, by telephone, and by referral from the community liaison nurse visiting at home.

Bladder care

Patients are taught the most effective method of bladder emptying (see pages 26-9 for long term bladder management). Although men with high tetraplegia can often tap over the bladder to induce a detrusor contraction, they will be unable to fit condoms and leg bags or empty their bags. People with high tetraplegia also cannot make drinks for themselves and will require help in maintaining a high fluid intake. In women with high tetraplegia the bladder is normally best managed by an indwelling catheter. The alternative of having to be transferred on and off the toilet every two to four hours, and probably also being constantly wet, is not acceptable. Self intermittent catheterisation is the best method for most women with paraplegia and some with low tetraplegia, and also for an appreciable number of men. It is particularly successful in patients with an acontractile bladder.

Urinary tract infections are common but reduced by adequate hydration and often by urinary acidification. In general antibiotics are given only when an infection causes systemic symptoms.

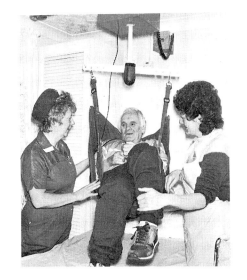

District nurse and care attendant using an electric hoist at home.

Nutrition and bowel care

Patients with spinal cord injury, particularly those with high lesions, are often unable to exercise adequately and are prone to excessive weight gain, which can further limit their mobility and independence. In the long term, most patients tend to be constipated and will benefit from dietary re-education. A high fibre diet of good nutritional standard, but with a controlled calorific content, is important. Care needs to be taken in changing the diet if constipation, or more seriously diarrhoea with the risk of bowel accidents, are to be avoided. In practice most patients evacuate their bowels daily or on alternate days. Where possible, the timing and frequency of bowel evacuation should be made to fit in with the person's chosen lifestyle. The relationships between mother and son and, particularly, between young wife and husband are such that they may find it difficult to attend to bowels. If help is needed, assistance from the district nurse may be requested.

Tetraplegic and paraplegic patients with upper motor neurone cord lesions have reflex bowel activity, and evacuation can usually be produced by inserting glycerine suppositories or by anal digital stimulation, or both. Patients with high tetraplegia or frail patients may have to be lifted or hoisted on to the toilet, but many have insufficient balance to permit this, and in these circumstances bowel evacuation will have to take place on the bed with the patient in the lateral position.

Patients with low paraplegia with a lower motor neurone cord lesion will have a flaccid bowel and will need to evacuate their bowel manually or by straining using the abdominal muscles, or by a combination of the two methods. They should be able to transfer themselves or be transferred on to a toilet with a padded seat to prevent pressure sores from prolonged sitting.

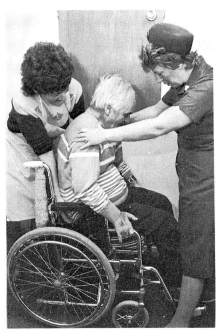

Care attendant and district nurse positioning tetraplegic man in his wheelchair.

Patients with paraplegia or low tetraplegia can learn how to transfer into and out of bed, a shower or bath, and a car, but those with high tetraplegia have to be lifted or hoisted.

Autonomic dysreflexia is commonly associated with bladder or bowel pathology, particularly overdistension. By the time of discharge from hospital, patients should be fully aware of the signs and symptoms of autonomic dysreflexia and be able to direct people to help find and remove the cause.

Further educational principles are described in the chapter on nursing.

Teaching the family and community staff

By the time they are discharged from hospital patients should feel thoroughly responsible for their own care. The appropriate family members are invited to the spinal unit for individual instruction on how to assist with the patient's care, and also to attend a study day.

Transfer of care from hospital to community

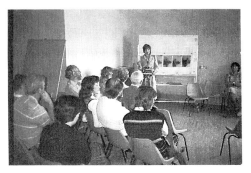

Teaching session for families, in which all disciplines participate.

As spinal cord injury is uncommon, district nurses and general practitioners may not have cared for such patients before. District nurses and care attendants are invited to the spinal unit to work with the patients' primary care teams and learn specific aspects of care for their prospective patients. They are also invited to attend study days to receive tuition in pressure sore prevention, bladder and bowel management, aids to daily living, and psychological and long term aspects of spinal cord injury. In our experience almost all those community staff invited welcome the opportunity to visit the unit. The community liaison nurse also visits community staff in their areas and will advise on request.

Preparation for discharge from hospital

> **Providers of care**
>
> Family
>
> District nurses
>
> Care attendants
>
> Resident carers/personal assistants
>
> —privately employed
>
> —employed by disabled person using state
>   benefits

> **Care attendant schemes**
>
> National Health Service (NHS)
>
> Social services
>
> NHS social services joint funded
>
> Leonard Cheshire Foundation
>   family support services

> **Community case conference**
>
> *Spinal unit*
> Primary nurse
> Social worker
> Occupational
>   therapist
> Community
>   liaison nurse
>
> *Community*
> District nurse
> Community nurse
>   manager
> Social worker
> Occupational therapist
> Home care organiser
> General practitioner

Who provides the care?

The care outlined implies a large time input, and for patients with high tetraplegia this has to be given by other people. Who is to provide this care? The obvious answer is the family. However, it is unusual if the family can, or should be expected to, provide sole care for a highly dependent person for a lifetime. Traditionally, care for such people has been a choice between family or an institution, but many very disabled people wish to maintain their independence as much as possible and live in the place of their choice. Outside help from the community will be necessary to achieve this goal. Increasing numbers of people with high level tetraplegia choose to set up their own home by employing personal assistants.

The community case conference

The resources available in the community for a particular patient are identified from the spinal centre by the social worker and community liaison nurse. Patients and their relatives must be kept fully informed so that correct decisions are made regarding their care in the community. Community case conferences held in the patients' home areas can be useful by enabling patients and their families to meet community and spinal unit staff to plan effectively for all aspects of future care needs. It also means that all interested parties can meet each other to exchange information on a patient's future care. A flexible approach is necessary as the problems vary greatly from patient to patient.

Many patients with spinal cord injury are young people who before their injury were in the process of making decisions about their lives. Immediately after such a catastrophic injury, and often for several years afterwards, they find it difficult to make major decisions such as where to live, with whom, who is best to assist with their care, and what to do about their job. Sometimes a temporary solution is necessary, and allowance should be made for the possibility of later change.

Planning for discharge home

The case conference can also be used to plan maximum help for the patients and their families initially, as the months after discharge are physically and emotionally exhausting for both. When patients with high care needs go home from hospital without any help from outside the family the pressure is often too great, and a breakdown of family relationships is likely. Patients are faced with the harsh reality of everyday living, without the support and protection of a spinal injuries unit, and should accept maximum help initially. Providing help to allow the family members to have time for themselves is of primary importance, otherwise resentment at being tied for 24 hours a day will build up, along with physical and emotional exhaustion.

Skills required for independent living

- Interviewing, employing, and training staff
- Managing personal finances

Interim care facilities

Young disabled unit
   (health or social services)

Leonard Cheshire home

Local hospital

Referring hospital

Respite care

Sessions every week

Fixed periods when disabled person goes to
   young disabled unit, Cheshire home, etc

Spinal Injuries Association personal assistant
   to home for 1-2 weeks

Disabled person on holiday with volunteer
   group or care attendant/personal assistant

Transfer from hospital to community eased by:

Single and joint visits from:

District nurse (once a day initially)

Care attendant (twice a day)

Community liaison nurse from spinal unit
   (within a month after discharge from
   hospital, thereafter on request)

Planning for independent living

Many tetraplegic people choose to live independently when discharged from the spinal unit. The community nurses and social services may provide information about statutory care facilities in patients' home areas. These services, however, are often unable to meet fully the care needs of someone with a high level injury and may need to be supplemented. Many young people prefer to employ a personal assistant, to live in or nearby, to help with personal care and daily living activities. This allows people to be "in charge" of their lives but requires them to develop skills in interviewing, finance management, and teaching. When financial compensation for the injury is not available, people may contact their local social services and health authorities for financial support, along with the benefits listed on page 44. Assistance in funding, advertising, and writing contracts may be obtained from centres for independent living. Initially, people choosing this option often require additional support from the spinal unit and community nurses, as they very quickly become totally responsible for their own care on leaving hospital.

Planning for interim care and respite care

When their homes have not been adapted for wheelchair use before patients' discharge from hospital, interim care may be necessary and can help to act as a bridge between the protection of a spinal injuries unit and the harsh reality of everyday living.

Respite care planned before discharge can be a valuable provision to help prevent a breakdown in relationships with families or carers.

Easing transfer from hospital to community

The support of the district nursing service is often invaluable in easing the transfer from hospital to the community. Before discharge patients will have had some weekends at home. Difficulties experienced by them and their families can be discussed with the district nurse, who can assess the situation and contact the spinal unit if advice is required. The families are often reassured to know that there is an effective link between the hospital and community. To maintain this link the initial discharge plan may require a district nurse each morning to provide nursing care with help from either a care attendant or family member. The families would then be alone until the evening, when a care attendant could come in to help undress the patient and help him or her into bed. It is also important for patients and families to be able to get out of the house, possibly with the help of a care attendant. The system of care can change as the family, patient, and care attendant become more confident and as the district nurse teaches and supports them to take on more skilled tasks. The district nurse might then provide only occasional check visits.

The early weeks at home

However well a patient's community care is planned, problems may still arise. For this reason all patients are visited by the community liaison nurse from the spinal unit within a month of discharge, and at other times as required at the request of the patient, family, carers, district nurse, or general practitioner. Community liaison nurses will also visit community staff in their areas and visit patients jointly with them to both educate and further assist in the transfer of care from hospital to home.

LATER MANAGEMENT AND COMPLICATIONS—I

David Grundy, Anthony Tromans

Spinal deformity

Predisposing factors
- Age at injury
- Level of lesion
- Completeness of lesion
- Inadequate treatment of bony injury
- Laminectomy without stabilisation and fusion
- Gross leg deformities

Preventing spinal deformity is extremely important, particularly as correcting an established deformity may be difficult and potentially hazardous if major surgery is necessary.

The most important factors predisposing to spinal deformity are the age at injury and the level and completeness of the cord lesion. The growing child is most at risk of developing a major spinal deformity, usually scoliosis. The higher the neurological level and the more complete the lesion, the greater the tendency to spinal deformity. Inadequate early treatment of the bony injury or inappropriate surgical exploration by laminectomy without stabilisation and fusion may also lead to late deformity. Leg deformities may also affect the spine—for instance, flexion contractures of the hips cause pelvic obliquity and excessive lumbar lordosis, and if the deformity is asymmetrical scoliosis will result.

In children spinal bracing is required until vertebral growth is completed, and until then periods of sitting should be limited. An erect frame such as a swivel walker and a prone trolley to limit sitting in a wheelchair are helpful, particularly in the very young. In adults with thoracolumbar injury bracing is often advisable even if internal fixation has been performed. Spinal deformity severe enough to require surgical correction requires careful preoperative assessment, respiratory complications being a particular hazard of the operation.

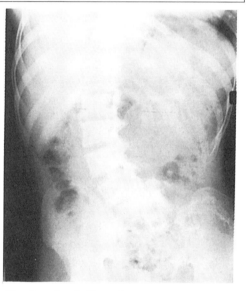

Late scoliotic deformity in an 18 year old after inadequate treatment of L4-5 fracture-dislocation four years earlier.

Pathological fractures

Although internal fixation of limb fractures sustained at the time of the spinal cord injury may often be indicated, particularly to assist nursing, the emphasis later is on a more conservative approach. After injury to the spinal cord, bones in the paralysed limbs become osteoporotic, and pathological fractures may occur with minimal or even no obvious trauma. A common injury is supracondylar fracture of the femur caused by the patient falling out of the wheelchair on to his or her knees. Violent spasticity of the hip flexors, particularly if the leg rotates, can fracture the femoral shaft.

With rare exceptions treatment should be conservative. A well padded splint may be enough. If a circular cast is used it should be split, allowing the skin to be inspected daily for signs of pressure. Insufficient padding or failure to split a cast on a paralysed limb carries a high risk of producing pressure sores and painless ischaemia secondary to swelling. Immobilisation should not be prolonged as it is important to avoid joint stiffness, which might limit the patient's independence. Fortunately, fracture healing is usually satisfactory and callus formation good.

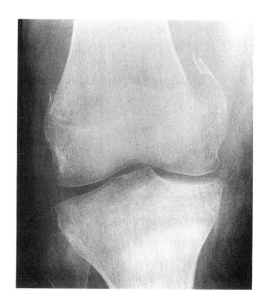

Supracondylar fracture of the right femur, the result of a "minor" fall in a patient with mid-thoracic paraplegia.

Post-traumatic syringomyelia (cystic myelopathy)

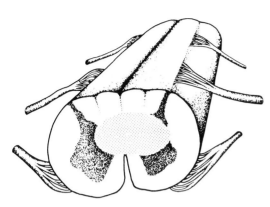

Common site of post-traumatic cavitation of the cord.

Post-traumatic syringomyelia, an ascending myelopathy due to secondary cavitation in the spinal cord, is seen in at least 2% of patients. Symptoms may appear as early as two months after injury or in rare instances be delayed for over 30 years, the average latent period having previously been reported as eight to nine years. The commonest presenting symptom is pain in the arm, usually unilateral, described as a dull ache but occasionally as burning or stabbing. The earliest sign is usually a dissociated sensory loss, with impaired or absent pain and temperature sensation (spinothalamic loss) and preservation of light touch and joint position sense (posterior column sparing). Some patients also have sensory loss over the face due to an extension of the cavitation into the upper cervical cord, which affects the spinal tract of the trigeminal nerve and, in rare instances, the brain stem. When present, motor loss is of a lower motor neurone type and is usually unilateral. Though there may be remissions, the condition may progress, perhaps even to the extent of converting low paraplegia into tetraplegia.

Though essentially clinical, the diagnosis is confirmed by magnetic resonance imaging (MRI) or computed tomography with myelography. Treatment is by surgical drainage of the syringomyelic cavity. Pain is usually relieved, but relief of sensory symptoms and motor loss is less predictable.

Pain

Factors contributing to chronic pain

- Inadequate early pain relief of the spinal injury
- Spinal malalignment
- Nerve root compression
- Incompleteness of spinal cord lesion
- Poor emotional adjustment

Treatment of chronic pain

- Treat spinal instability and nerve root compression
- Distraction by busy rehabilitation programme
- Antidepressants/antipsychotics, eg amitriptyline-perphenazine combination
- Anticonvulsants, eg carbamazepine
- Transcutaneous nerve stimulation
- Acupuncture
- Hypnotherapy and relaxation techniques
- Spinal cord stimulation

    (Analgesics relatively ineffective)

    (Surgical techniques have little place)

In the acute stage after spinal cord injury the choice of analgesic may be difficult, especially in tetraplegic patients, in whom opioid analgesics (for example, morphine) may precipitate respiratory failure. They are, however, administered as a low dose constant infusion or by a patient controlled analgesia system (PCAS), the most satisfactory methods of controlling pain. The risks of respiratory depression are minimal once the correct dosage has been calculated.

Chronic intractable pain after spinal cord injury is a particularly difficult problem, largely because of the profound emotional effect of a severe disability occurring suddenly and unexpectedly in a previously healthy and often young patient. A self generating mechanism has been suggested for pain in the central nervous system, and it is possible, particularly in patients with incomplete spinal cord lesions, that abnormal sensations arising adjacent to the site of cord damage will act as stimuli for the subsequent development of chronic pain. The "conditioning" effect of early acute pain on the nervous system can be minimised by a sympathetic attitude towards the patient and prompt administration of adequate doses of analgesics to relieve pain from the site of bony injury. The spine should be realigned, nerve root compression relieved if necessary, and the limbs correctly positioned and regularly put through a full range of passive movements.

During the first few weeks or months after injury discomfort or pain may occur, which appears to be related to neural damage rather than the musculoskeletal trauma. It may take one of several forms. There may be an unpleasant or painful sensation in a paralysed area similar to the phantom phenomenon experienced after amputation. Another example is an acute burning or stabbing sensation felt immediately below the neurological level of the lesion or several segments distally, which can be continuous and extremely incapacitating. This type of pain is often seen in cauda equina lesions. The pain of the incomplete lesion is also a burning sensation associated with hyperalgesia and may be increased by peripheral stimulation or movement of the limb. Pain that follows an anatomical distribution at or just below the level of the cord lesion may be due to damage at the root entry zone, but in these circumstances it is important to exclude nerve root compression, which may rarely require surgical decompression.

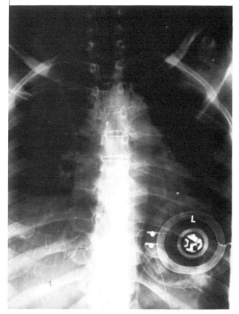

Dorsal column stimulator, sometimes helpful in treating chronic pain. By courtesy of Dr Lee Illis, Wessex Neurological Centre.

A considerable number of patients complain of severe chronic pain, and many others are aware of abnormal sensation below the level of the lesion. Continuing spinal instability must be treated, but otherwise mobilisation should begin as early as possible after injury, the distraction of full participation in a busy rehabilitation programme being the most helpful measure.

Analgesics do not satisfactorily relieve pain associated with neural damage, but tricyclic antidepressants combined with phenothiazines or carbamazepine sometimes help, and transcutaneous nerve stimulation acupuncture, relaxation techniques, and hypnotherapy may give relief. Spinal cord (dorsal column) stimulation has been used in a few centres with some success, probably by interrupting the ascending pain pathways and releasing endogenous endorphins. However, surgical techniques such as posterior rhizotomy and spinothalamic tractotomy, although interrupting the pain pathways, have little place because, even if pain is relieved, the effect may be short lasting. Dorsal root entry zone coagulation, successful in controlling the severe pain of root avulsion injuries, has been disappointing in its effect on pain after spinal cord injury.

Sexual function

Spinal cord centres for sexual function

Erection	Reflex	Parasympathetic S2, 3, 4 (nervi erigentes)
	Psychogenic	Sympathetic T11 to L2 (hypogastric nerve)
Emission		Sympathetic T11 to L2 (hypogastric nerve)
Ejaculation		Somatic S2, 3, 4 (pudendal nerve)

Sexual function depends on the level and completeness of the spinal cord lesion. If the lesion is incomplete sexual function may be affected to a varying degree and sometimes not at all. In women, although there is often an initial period of amenorrhoea after spinal cord injury, fertility is unimpaired. In men with complete or substantial spinal cord lesions, the ability to achieve normal erections, ejaculate, and father children can be greatly disturbed.

Erections

Most patients with complete upper motor neurone lesions of the cord have reflex, but not psychogenic, erections. However, the erections are not always sustained or strong enough for sexual intercourse. In patients with complete lower motor neurone lesions parasympathetic connections from the S2 to S4 segments of the cord to the corpora cavernosa are interrupted, so that reflex erections are usually impossible.

Difficulty in achieving a satisfactory erection can often be overcome using intracavernous papaverine injections or vacuum erection aids and a compressive retainer ring. Insertion of a penile implant is also possible, but carries a small risk of infection or erosion of the implant, which if it occurs will necessitate its removal. Some men with a sacral anterior nerve root stimulator are able to achieve stimulator-driven erections, in addition to using the stimulator primarily for micturition.

Emission and ejaculation

For seminal emission to occur the sympathetic outflow from T11 to L2 segments of the cord to the vasa deferentia, seminal vesicles, and prostate must be intact. Emission infers a trickling emission of semen, with no rhythmic contractions of the pelvic floor muscles as in true ejaculation. Some patients with complete cord lesions at lumbar or sacral level may have both psychogenic erections and emissions.

If ejaculation is not possible by natural means, it may be induced by direct stimulation of the fraenum of the penis using a vibrator. If this is unsuccessful, electroejaculation may produce what is actually an emission.

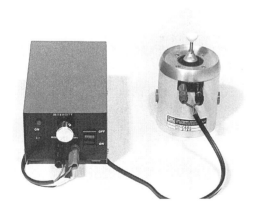

Ling 201 vibrator, for inducing seminal emission by penile stimulation.

In men who cannot ejaculate using the vibrator, or where electroejaculation is difficult, a hypogastric plexus stimulator can be implanted to obtain seminal emission, using a single inductive link across the skin. There is a risk of autonomic dysreflexia in patients with a lesion above T6 during these procedures.

For men who can achieve neither emission nor ejaculation, spermatozoa can be collected in implanted reservoirs connected to the vas deferentia and retrieved by transcutaneous aspiration.

Preparation for sexual intercourse

Preparation for sexual intercourse includes ensuring that the bladder is as empty as possible. A man with an indwelling catheter should preferably remove it, but it may be strapped back on to the shaft of the penis. In the woman a catheter may be left in situ. The ablebodied partner tends to be the more active, and this has a bearing on the positions used for intercourse.

Men with lesions above T6 are at risk of autonomic dysreflexia developing during ejaculation. If this occurs intercourse should be curtailed, the man sat upright, and if necessary given sublingual nifedipine or glyceryl trinitrate.

Fertility

Fertility is generally reduced in men after spinal cord injury. The sperm count is usually low, with diminished motility due to various factors, probably including continuing non-ejaculation, raised testicular temperature, and infection. The quality of the seminal fluid tends to improve with repeated ejaculations, however, and successful insemination has been reported both with the vibrator and by electroejaculation. Brindley previously estimated that over 20% of paraplegic and tetraplegic men should be fertile using these techniques. However, the success rate has recently improved with the use of assisted conception techniques, including enhancement of seminal fluid, intrauterine insemination, and assisted reproductive technology, such as in vitro fertilisation (IVF) and gamete intrafallopian transfer (GIFT).

Labour

If the spinal cord lesion is complete above T10, labour may be painless and forceps delivery required because of inability to bear down effectively during the second stage of labour. Autonomic dysreflexia during labour is a risk in patients with lesions at T6 and above, but this complication can be prevented by epidural anaesthesia.

Fulfilment in relationships

It should be emphasised that emotional and psychological factors are as important as physical factors in a satisfying relationship and that such a relationship is possible even after severe spinal cord injury. This needs reiterating, particularly to young men who are otherwise apt to see their altered sexual function as a profound loss. Although sensation in the sexual organs may be reduced or absent, imaginative use can be made of touching and caressing, as areas of the body above the level of the spinal cord lesion may develop heightened sensation as erogenous zones. Some couples find that the extra time and effort required for sexual expression after one of them has suffered a spinal cord injury enriches their lives and results in a more understanding and caring relationship.

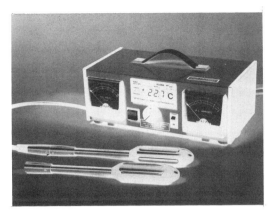

Seager electroejaculation unit with different sized rectal probes.

Aids to sexual function and fulfilment in relationships

To enhance sexual expression

Use imagination, time, and effort in touching parts of the body not affected by the injury, exploring both partners' preferences, experimenting with other erotic stimuli, etc.

For erection

Intracavernous papaverine injection
Vacuum erection aid and compressive retainer ring
Penile implant (small risk of infection)
Sacral anterior nerve root stimulator

For ejaculation or seminal emission

Vibrator
Electroejaculation unit
Hypogastric plexus stimulator

To collect spermatozoa

Implant reservoirs connected to vas deferentia and
Retrieve collected spermatozoa by transcutaneous aspiration

Further assisted conception techniques

Seminal fluid enhancement
Intrauterine insemination
In vitro fertilisation
Gamete intrafallopian transfer

To counteract autonomic dysreflexia (possible in men during ejaculation, in women during labour, if lesion above T6)

Sublingual nifedipine or glyceryl trinitrate

LATER MANAGEMENT AND COMPLICATIONS—II

David Grundy, Anthony Tromans

Psychological factors

Factors

- Acute stage—sensory deprivation, most noticeable in high lesions
  —swings in mood: fear, anger, depression, euphoria, frustration
- Later stages—long period of adjustment required (2-3 years)
  —continuing support necessary

The initial psychological adjustment to a spinal cord injury has already been discussed, but long term support may also be required. The frustrations associated with the physical limitations of such a severe injury are compounded by the fact that most patients are young and before injury led active lives, often expressing themselves mainly through physical activities. The sudden inability to continue in this manner and the need to lead a more ordered life can mean a very difficult and prolonged period of adjustment. Failure to recognise that this process can continue for as long as two or three years may damage the process of rehabilitation and the patient's ultimate resettlement. The patient needs time to come to terms with his or her new status and to make decisions about the future without undue pressure. Continuing support will be needed after discharge from hospital, both from community services and from outpatient visits, and the problems and fears of ablebodied partners or close relatives must also be remembered.

The hand in tetraplegia

Aims

- To restore active elbow extension
- To provide a functional grip
- To improve manual dexterity

Factors in selection for surgery

Absolute prerequisites

- Neurological level below C5
- No change in muscle power for at least 6 months
- Well motivated patient

Relative factors in selection

- Adequate sensation in hand
- Minimal or no spasticity
- Minimal or no contractures

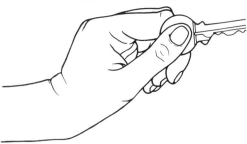

Key grip, achieved by using the Moberg technique.

Most tetraplegic patients give priority to restoring function in their arms. In selected patients with injuries below the fifth cervical segment surgery may be helpful, the main aims being to restore active elbow extension and a functional hand grip. An important factor in patient selection is motivation, as treatment will be prolonged, requiring perseverance and cooperation from the patient. The timing of surgery is important, and the neurological deficit should have been stable for at least six months. The lack of normal sensation is not a contraindication, but contractures, joint deformity, and spasticity require prior treatment by splintage, therapy, or surgery and will often be deleterious to the outcome.

Restoring elbow extension by transferring the posterior third of the deltoid muscle into the triceps tendon enables a patient to reach overhead and also facilitates wheelchair skills, lifting to relieve pressure, and transferring.

Functional hand grip may be restored with a passive flexor tenodesis, once active wrist extension is achieved, by transferring the brachioradialis into the insertion of the radial extensors. If wrist extension is active and the extensor carpi radialis longus or brachioradialis are normally innervated, they may be transferred into the flexor digitorum profundus to achieve finger flexion or into the flexor pollicis longus for thumb flexion.

A passive key grip, as described by Moberg, is possible during wrist extension by tenodesing the flexor pollicis longus to the lower end of the radius and stabilising the interphalangeal joint. With the wrist extended the thumb will then oppose the radial side of the index finger.

Further surgical procedures may be used to achieve an intrinsic balance and improve hand function in lower cervical injuries.

Functional electrical stimulation

Aims

- Leg—to augment, or dispense with, conventional calipers
  —to restore walking in patients who otherwise would not be able to walk using conventional calipers

- Arm—to re-establish hand grip

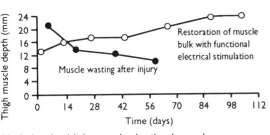

Variation in thigh muscle depth, shown by ultrasound. Note rapid muscle wasting after injury, which can be restored by functional electrical stimulation.

In recent years there has been renewed interest in the role of functional electrical stimulation (FES) of paralysed muscles to provide arm function in tetraplegia and restore walking in paraplegia. In a few patients it has been possible to dispense with conventional calipers and establish an effective gait. Functional electrical stimulation also reduces muscle wasting, improves leg circulation, and may minimise osteoporosis. Stimulation is more difficult if there is a lower motor neurone lesion, when its functional applications are limited.

The stimulation programme is protracted, and a graduated daily training programme of isometric contractions to strengthen the muscles is required. Standing involving the stimulation of multiple muscle groups (quadriceps, peroneals, and possibly the glutei) may often be achieved in three months, the control of balance being facilitated by feedback from joint position sensors. Once standing has been achieved, attempts to restore walking may be made. Functional electrical stimulation may also be combined with orthotic devices such as the hip guidance orthosis or the reciprocating gait orthosis.

Research continues on the stimulation of forearm muscles to re-establish hand grip in tetraplegia in cases where tendon transfer surgery may be inadequate, but its use may be limited or impossible because there is often an element of lower motor neurone loss in cervical cord injuries due to anterior horn cell damage.

As yet functional electrical stimulation has not been fully developed or adequately assessed, and until its long term effects on joints and other physiological responses have been evaluated its use should probably be limited to a few centres.

Prognosis

Age at injury (years)	Life expectancy (years)	Relative mortality
Incomplete tetraplegia		
20	44	
30	36	2·09×expected mortality
40	27	in normal population
50	18	
Complete tetraplegia		
20	30	
30	23	7·67×expected mortality
40	15	in normal population
50	9	
Incomplete paraplegia		
20	46	
30	37	1·86×expected mortality
40	28	in normal population
50	19	
Complete paraplegia		
20	40	
30	32	3·18×expected mortality
40	23	in normal population
50	15	

Table adapted from Geisler WO, Jousse AT, Wynne-Jones M, Breithaupt D. Survival in traumatic spinal cord injury. *Paraplegia* 1983;**21**:364-73 and based on calculations made in 1980 by actuarial department of Manufacturers Life Insurance Company, Toronto.

It is important to indicate the probable degree of recovery at an early stage to both patient and relatives, to make planning for the future realistic. The question of financial compensation will often arise in accident cases, and an informed opinion will be required on the degree of functional recovery that is likely and the effect on life expectancy.

Recovery after a complete cord lesion is far less likely than after an incomplete lesion, but it is unwise to predict non-recovery too early, as some patients with an incomplete injury may initially appear to be totally paralysed because of spinal cord oedema and contusion, which later resolves.

Forecasting the outcome in patients with an incomplete lesion is notoriously difficult. Too optimistic a prognosis may lead to great disappointment, with loss of morale and decreased interest in rehabilitation when hopes are unfulfilled. Contrary to a widely held view, however, neurological improvement can be seen later than two years after injury, not only with nerve root and cauda equina lesions but also with cord injuries.

Mortality in acutely injured patients managed in a spinal injuries unit is now less than 5%. Death within the first few days is likely to be from respiratory failure, particularly in high tetraplegia. The presence of multiple injuries, age, and previous health of the patient all play a part. In patients surviving the period immediately after injury pulmonary embolism is the commonest cause of death in the acute phase.

With the modern management of spinal cord injury, life expectancy has improved over recent years; as a consequence atherosclerosis and its complications are now a major cause of late death, but renal failure still figures prominently, as does respiratory tract infection in tetraplegic patients.

Conclusions

Useful addresses

The Disability Alliance Educational and Research
  Association, Universal House,
88-94 Wentworth Street, London E1 7SA
071 247 8776
Provides advice about welfare benefits

Disabled Living Foundation,
380-384 Harrow Road, London W9 2HU
071 289 6111
An information centre with an extensive display of
equipment

The Association to aid the Sexual and Personal
  Relationships of People with a Disability (SPOD),
286 Camden Road, London N7 OBJ
071 607 8851
Deals with sexual problems connected with all types
of disability. Helpful series of leaflets

Spinal Injuries Association, Newpoint House,
76 St James's Lane, London N10 3DF
081 444 2121
The association for spinal cord injured people and all
involved in their care. Excellent quarterly newsletter

Great progress has been made in the care of patients with spinal cord injuries since the 1940s, when spinal injuries units were first established. There has been a remarkable decrease in complications using the multidisciplinary approach provided by such units, yet some patients are still denied referral. Unless complete recovery occurs, patients should have lifelong hospital outpatient follow up but with emphasis on continuing care and support in the community.

Although it is right to be optimistic about the future of these patients, their injuries can make a devastating change to their lives. In many cases the injuries need not have happened. For example, a high proportion of road traffic accidents are caused by alcohol consumption, high speeds, and dangerous driving, motorcyclists being particularly vulnerable. Ignorance of the danger of diving into shallow water results in many injuries to the cervical spine. Failure to take simple precautions in the home, such as ensuring that stairs are adequately lit at night for the elderly, may result in falls with cervical hyperextension injuries. Carelessness in contact sports can lead to serious injury. Recognition of this fact has led responsible authorities such as the Rugby Football Union to modify the laws of the game and issue advice on how it can be made safer, but much more could be done in other aspects of accident prevention.

Finally, those who work with patients with spinal cord injuries are often impressed by the surprisingly high quality of life possible after injury. Many achieve a remarkable a degree of independence, earn their own living, choose to marry, have children, and participate fully in family life. They may indeed have special qualities because they have successfully come to terms with their disability, and many will make a valuable contribution to society.

We thank the Department of Medical Photography, Odstock Hospital, Salisbury, and the Department of Medical Illustration, Charing Cross Hospital, London, for the photographs, and Amanda German, Department of Medical Illustration, Charing Cross Hospital for the line drawings and Mary Grundy for checking the text and reading the proofs.

Further reading

Bedbrook GM, ed. *The care and mangement of spinal cord injuries*. New York: Springer-Verlag, 1981. A guide to medical management of the spinal cord injured patient.

Bedbrook GM, ed. *Lifetime care of the paraplegic patient*. Edinburgh: Churchill Livingstone, 1985. A comprehensive textbook on the long term aspects of care, written by and for a multidisciplinary team.

Bloch R, Bashaum M, eds. *Management of spinal injuries*. Baltimore: Williams and Wilkins, 1986. Offers excellent in-depth resource material on a wide variety of topics.

Bromley I. *Tetraplegia and paraplegia—a guide for physiotherapists*. 4th ed. Endinburgh: Churchill Livingstone, 1991. Particularly relevant for therapists, with many clear illustrations.

Fallon B. *So you're paralysed*. London: Spinal Injuries Association, 1975. Written for the newly paralysed patient, but useful for everyone concerned in the long term management of spinal cord injury.

Ford JR, Duckworth B. *Physical management for the quadriplegic patient*. 2nd ed. Philadelphia: FA Davis Company, 1987. A well illustrated handbook for occupational therapists.

Leyson JF. *Sexual rehabilitation of the spinal cord injured patient*. New Jersey: Humana Press, 1991. Very good cover of all aspects of sexuality.

Meyer PR, ed. *Surgery of spine trauma*. New York: Churchill Livingstone, 1989. Includes a comprehensive account of the mechanisms and management of the bony and soft tissue injury.

Morris J, ed. *Able lives*. London: The Women's Press Ltd., 1989. A good account of women's experience of paralysis.

Rogers Michael A. *Living with paraplegia*. London: Faber and Faber, 1986. Excellent practical advice for paraplegics, tetraplegics, and their families, written from experience.

Trieschmann RB. *Spinal cord injuries— psychological, social and vocational rehabilitation*. 2nd ed. New York: Demos, 1988. The only book devoted exclusively to the psychosocial impact of spinal cord injury on disabled individuals.

Vinken PJ, Bruyn GW, eds. *Injuries of the spine and spinal cord*. Amsterdam: North Holland, 1976. (Handbook of Clinical Neurology Series parts 25 and 26.) A comprehensive and authorative reference book.

Whiteneck G, Adler C, Carter R E, Lammertse D P, Manley S, Menter R, eds. *The management of high quadriplegia*. New York: Demos, 1989. A comprehensive guide to all aspects of management of high lesion patients.

Zejdlik CM. *Management of spinal cord injury*. Monterey: Wordsworth Health Sciences Division, 1983. A practical and comprehensive textbook for nurses.

Directory for disabled people. Compiled by Ann Darnbrough, Derek Kinrade. 5th ed. Cambridge: Woodhead-Faulkner, 1988. A comprehensive handbook of information and opportunities for disabled and handicapped people.

Disability rights handbook. London: Disability Alliance, published annually. Provides information about welfare benefits and the obligations of statutory authorities.

INDEX

α Adrenergic blocker   27
Abdominal
  binder   19, 38
  distension   5, 16
  injuries   5
  muscles   36, 47
  reflex   5
  straining   27
Abscess, periurethral   16, 24
Accident
  conscious patient   3
  evacuation from   1, 4
  management at scene of   2–3
  prevention   55
  transfer to hospital from   4
  unconscious patient   2–3
Accident and emergency department, nursing
    management   31
Activities of daily living   41–2
Acupuncture   51, 52
Adjustment, psychological   30, 43, 45, 54
Aids to daily living (ADL)   30, 48
Air evacuation   18
Airway patency   2
Alcohol in intrathecal block   23
Amenorrhoea   52
Amitriptyline   51
Anaesthetist   12
Anal fissure   35
Anal reflex   5, 6
Analgesia   3, 51, 52
Anger   30
Ankylosing spondylitis   9
Anorexia   34
Anterior cord syndrome   6
Anterior horn cell damage   55
Antibiotic use   18, 25, 28, 47
Anticholinergic drugs, and bladder   25
Anticoagulation   17
Anticonvulsants   51
Antidepressants   51, 52
Antipsychotics   51
Anxiety   30
Aortic dissection   10
Aortography   10
Aperients   35
Areflexia   3
Arm
  care 31, 33
  function   55
Arthritis, septic   23
Artificial urinary sphincter (AUS)   29
Ascorbic acid, urine acidification   26
Assisted conception techniques   53
Assisted coughing   36
Ataxia   6
Atelectasis   12
Atherosclerosis   55
Atlantoaxial dislocation   20
Atlantoaxial fusion   21
Atlantoaxial subluxation   9
Atlas   9
Atropine   13
Attendance allowance   44
Autonomic dysreflexia   47, 53
  causes   28, 47
  effects   28
  treatment   28, 47
Axial spondylolisthesis   21

Baclofen   23
Balance   37, 55
Beds
  Egerton   17, 31
  King's Fund   31
  profiling   19, 31, 37
Benefits, financial   44, 45
Bethanechol   27
Bladder
  acontractile   16, 25, 27, 28, 29, 47
  and sexual intercourse   53
  augmentation   27, 28, 29
  calculi   16, 24, 25, 26
  capacity   27, 28
  contractile   27, 28, 29
  distension   16, 24, 28, 34
  outlet obstruction   25, 27
  washout   16, 25, 28
Bladder management   24–9, 34–5, 46, 47, 48,
    53
  aims   24
  drugs   25, 26, 27
  long term   27
  men   26–7, 47
  nursing care   34–5
  women   28, 35, 47
Bladder neck
  incision   27, 28
  obstruction   27
Blankets   4
Blood pressure instability   30
Body image   30
Bone
  grafting   22
  growth in children   39
  heterotopic   22
Bowel management   35
  community   46, 47, 48
  manual evacuation   35
Brachioradialis   54
Bracing   22
  children   39, 50
Bradycardia   3, 13, 28, 33
Brain stem and syringomyelia   51
Breath, technology control by   42
Breathing exercises   12
Bronchoscopy   12
Brown-Séquard syndrome   6
Bulbocavernosus reflex   5, 6
Bupivacaine   23
Buprenorphine   3

Calculi
  bladder   16, 24, 25, 26
  renal   26
  ureteric   26
Calipers   38, 39, 55 *See also* Skull calipers
Carbachol   27
Carbamazepine   51, 52
Cardiac arrest   3, 13
Cardiovascular complications   13
Care attendants   31, 48, 49
Careers guidance   45
Caring for People   43
Case conference before hospital discharge   48
Catheterisation *See* Urinary catheterisation
Catheters
  blockage   28
  encrustation   16

indwelling   34, 37, 53
  latex   16, 25
  silicone   16, 25
  silver   25
  suprapubic   16, 28, 34, 35
Cauda equina lesions   6, 17, 25, 27, 51
  neurological recovery   13, 55
Central cord syndrome   6
Central nervous system pain   51
Centres for independent living   49
Cervical cord injuries   1, 2, 3, 4, 12, 13–5, 28
  high   12, 19
  hyperextension   2, 6, 9, 15
  operative fusion   15
  radiological investigations   7–11, 19
  respiratory complications   34
  skull traction   13–5, 19, 20, 21
  unstable   10, 15, 19, 20, 31
  upper   14, 20–1
Cervical ligamentous complex injuries   9, 19
  Cervical spinal cord blood supply   13
  Cervical spine positions   19
  extension   10, 19
  flexion   10, 19
  flexion-rotation   20
  neutral   19
Cervical spondylosis   6, 9, 15
Cervicothoracic junction   8, 20, 21
Cheshire Foundation (homes), Leonard   48, 49
Chest
  complications   36
  injuries   3, 5, 12, 17
  physiotherapy   36
Children
  physical rehabilitation   39
  spinal deformity   39, 50
  traction injury   9
  walking aids   39, 50
Chin lift   2, 31
Circulation   55
Clothing   46
Collars   2, 4, 19, 20, 31
Community care   46–9
  who provides   48–9
Community charge benefit   44
Community liaison nurse   46, 48, 49
Community support   44
Compensation, financial   44, 49
Compression
  bony   22
  cord   2
Computed tomogram   11
Computer technology   42
Condom drainage   24, 27, 47
Cone caliper   14
Constipation   35, 47
Continence   27, 29, 35
Contractures   17, 18, 23, 38
  hand   40, 54
Conus medullaris lesions   6, 25, 27
Coping mechanisms   30
Corticospinal tracts   5, 6
Coughing: assisted   12, 36
Counselling   44
Cranial nerve function   5
Creatinine   25
Criminal assault   1
Crutches   38, 39
Crutchfield caliper   14

Index

Cushions 23, 41, 46
Cystometrography 25, 26
Cystoplasty 28, 29
Cystoscopy 25, 28
Cystourethrography 25, 26

Dantrolene sodium 23
Decision making 15, 30, 34, 48, 54
Decompression 22
Defecation 29
Deltoid 54
Denial 30
Department of Social Security 44, 45
Dependence 30
Depolarising agent 13
Depression 30, 34, 44
Dermatomes 5
Detrusor muscle 16, 25, 26, 27, 47
    hyperreflexia 24
Detrusor-sphincter
    dyssynergia 26, 27, 28, 29
    effects 27
Diaphragm 12, 16
Diaphragmatic respiration 3, 12
Diarrhoea 47
Diazepam 23
Dietary re-education 34
Disability employment adviser 42
Disability living allowance 44
Disability working allowance 44
Disabled people
    benefits available 44
    community care 46–9
    employment 45
    independence 46, 48
    self help groups 45
    services available 45
Disablement employment advisers
    (DEAs) 45
Disc 9, 11
Discharge from hospital 30, 43, 47, 48, 49
Dislocation
    cervical spine 8, 15
    thoracolumbar spine 15
Disodium etidronate 22
Distal urethral sphincter 26
Distigmine bromide 27
District nurse 47, 48, 49
Diverticulum, urethral 24
Diving accidents 1, 36
Domestic accidents 1
Domiciliary ventilation 42
Dopamine 13
Dorsal column stimulator 52
Dorsal root entry zone coagulation 52
Drowning: pulmonary complications 18

Education
    community staff 47–8, 49
    family 47–8, 49
    patient 30, 31, 34–5, 46–7, 49
Egerton turning and tilting bed 17, 31
Ejaculation 52–3
    autonomic dysreflexia 53
    spinal cord centres 52
Elbow extension surgery 52
Electrical stimulation, functional 55
Electroejaculation 52, 53
Ellik evacuator (bladder/catheter) 25, 28
Employment 45
Employment Service 45
Enteral feeding 34
Ephedrine 19
Epididymo-orchitis 24
Epidural anaestheia 28, 53
Equinous contracture 17
Erection 29, 52–3
Erogenous zones 53
Ethyl alcohol 23
Euphoria 30
Exercise 47
Extension 2, 9
Extensor carpi radialis longus 54

Facet dislocation of cervical spine 8, 10
Facetectomy 21
Family
    acceptance of prognosis 30
    adjustment 30
    informing 48
    providing care 48, 49
    relationships 48, 49
    respite care 49
    teaching 48
Family credit 44
Fear 30
Feeding aids 34
Femoral fractures 50
Feneley procedure 28
Fertility 52, 53
Fibreoptic instruments 3, 12
Finance 44, 49
Finger flexion restoration 54
Fingernails 34
Fistula, urethral 16, 24
Flaccidity 3, 5, 6, 13
    bowel 35, 47
Flexion 10
Flexor digitorum profundus 54
Flexor pollicis longus 54
Fluid balance in catheterisation 34
Fluid intake
    maintaining high 47
    restriction in intermittent
        catheterisation 16, 24, 47
Foley catheter 25, 27
Foot drop 17
Forceps delivery 53
Forearm muscles functional electrical
    stimulation 55
Fractures See also individual bones
    burst 13, 20
    cervical spine 8, 13–5, 19–21
    internal fixation 15, 18, 20, 50
    pathological 50
    posterior facet joints 10
    reduction 13–5, 21
Frustration 30, 54
Functional electrical stimulation (FES) 55

Gait
    descriptions 39
    expectations 39
    functional electrical stimulation 55
    re-education 38
Gamete intrafallopian transfer (GIFT) 53
Gardner-Wells caliper 13, 15
Gastric regurgitation 2
Gastrointestinal tract 16
    stress ulceration 18
General practitioners 48, 49
Gibbus 5
Glutei 55
Glyceryl trinitrate 28, 53
Glycopyrronium 13
Grieving 30
Guilt 30
Gunshot injuries 15

Haematoma 9, 10
Haemopneumothorax 12
Halo bracing 20, 21
Halo traction 15
Hand function/grip 27
    functional electrical stimulation 55
    improving/restoring 54, 55
    in tetraplegia 18, 40, 54
"Hangman's" fracture 21
Harrington rods 21
Head immobilisation 4
Head injuries 5, 17
Head tilt 31
Helicopter use 4, 18
Heparin 17
Heterotopic ossification 22
Hexamine 26
Hip

extension 36
guidance orthosis (HGO) 38, 39, 55
joint 33
Hoists 47
Home alterations 41, 44
Home visit for occupational therapy 41
Hospital discharge 30, 43, 46–9
Housing 44
Housing benefit 44
Hurdles, psychological and physical 30
Hydration 47
Hydronephrosis 27, 29
Hyperalgesia 51
Hypercalciuria 16
Hyperextension 2
Hyperkalaemia 13
Hypertension: autonomic dysreflexia 28
Hypnotherapy 51, 52
Hypogastric plexus stimulator 53
Hypotension 3, 13 See also Postural
    hypotension
Hypothermia 4, 31
Hypovolaemic shock 3, 13
Hypoxia 3

Ileal conduit 27
Ileocystoplasty 27
Ileus, paralytic 5, 16, 34
Image intensifier 15
Imipramine 25, 26, 27, 29
Immobilisation 20, 21
Immobiliser 4
Implanted pump 23
Implanted reservoir 23, 53
Income support 44
Incomplete lesion 5, 21, 29, 39
    pain 51
    functional electrical stimulation 55
    patterns 6
    sexual function 52
Incontinence 26, 28, 29
Independence 46, 47, 49
Independent Living Fund 43
Industrial accidents 1
Industrial disablement benefit 44
Indwelling urethral catheterisation 25, 28, 47
    fluid balance 34
    tetraplegia 28
Infection 53
Information to patient 30, 46–8
Infusion of analgesics 3, 51
Insemination 53
Instability, bony 19
Intercostal muscle paralysis 3, 12, 36
Interim care 49
Intermittent urethral catheterisation 16, 24
    fluid balance 34
Internal fixation 20
Interphalangeal joints 40, 54
Interspinous gap, increased 3, 5
Intracranial haemorrhage 28
Intrathecal baclofen 23
Intrathecal block 23
Intravenous fluids 16
    overinfusion 3, 13
Intravesical pressure 26, 27, 29
Intubation
    blind 2
    endotracheal 2, 12, 13
    nasotracheal 2
    orotracheal 2
Invalid care allowance 44
Invalidity benefit 44
In vitro fertilisation 53
Ischaemia 50
Ischial pressure 23, 37, 41
Isolation 30
Isometrics 55

Jaw thrust 2, 31
Jefferson fracture 20
Joint
    care 18, 36, 40

deformity, hand   54
   position sensors   55
Kendrick extrication device   4
Key grip   54
King's Fund bed   31

Labour   53
Lamina fracture   22
Laminectomy   22
   and late deformity   50
Leg bags   47
Legs
   deformities   50
   nursing care   33
Levels of lesions
   bony   5
   neurological   3, 5
Lifestyle   30, 43, 47
Life threatening injuries   2, 4
Lifting to relieve pressure   31, 37, 46, 47, 54
Lifts   4, 32
Ligaments   9, 10
Limb care   18, 33
Log roll turn   2, 5, 17, 31
Loneliness   30
Lordosis   15, 17, 19
Lumbar region   33
Lung
   clearance   36
   pre-existing disease   36
   ventilation-perfusion mismatch   12
   vital capacity   12

Magnetic resonance imaging   11, 51
Malnutrition   34
Manipulation of cervical spine   15
Manual bowel evacuation   35, 47
Mattresses   31, 46
Medical Research Council scale   5
Menstruation   34
Metacarpophalangeal joints   40
Methylprednisolone   18
Mirrors   34, 46
Moberg technique   54
Mobilisation   22
Mobilisation into wheelchair   19, 22, 30, 37
Mobility   47
Mood swings   30
Morphine   51
Mortality   4
Motor neurone bladder   27
Motor neurone lesions
   conversion, upper to lower   23
   lower   6, 13, 35, 47, 51, 52, 55
   upper   13, 22, 27, 35, 47, 52
Motor point injections   23
Mouth sticks   42
Multiple injuries   5, 16, 31
Muscle
   charting   36
   groups, nerve supply   5
   power   39
   strengthening   36, 37, 54
   transfer   54
   wasting   55
Muscles See individual muscles
Myelography   11, 51
Myelopathy, cystic   51
Myotomes   5

Naloxone   3
Narcotic   3, 51
Nasogastric aspiration   16
Nasotracheal intubation   2
Natal cleft   19, 35
National Health Service   48
Neck immobilisation   4, 19, 20, 21, 31
Neck roll   15, 17, 19
Nelaton catheter   16, 24, 25
Nerve roots
   avulsion   52
   compression   51

lesions   51
Neural canal   13
Neural damage pain   51, 52
Neurectomy   23
Neurogenic shock   13
Neurological
   deficit   54
   deterioration   20
   examination   5
   outcome   18
   recovery   39
   symptoms   10
NHS charges, relief   44
Nifedipine   28, 53
Non-paralysed muscle strengthening   36, 37
Non-steroidal anti-inflammatory
   drugs   3, 22
Nursing   30–5
   aims   30
   management   31
   organisation   30
Nutrition   37, 47

Occipital region pressure sores   15
Occupational therapy   40–2
Odontoid process   7, 9
   fractures   21
   radiological investigations   7
Oedema
   cord   12, 36, 55
   pulmonary   13
Opioid analgesic administration   51
Oropharyngeal airway   2
Orotracheal intubation   2
Orthotic aids   38, 39, 55
Ossification, heterotopic   22
Osteoporosis   38, 50, 55
Oswestry standing frame   38
Overdistraction   21
Overinfusion   2, 13
Oxybutynin   25, 27
Oxygen   2

Pain   2, 15–2
   during flexion-extension radiographs   20
   sensation   6
Pancuronium   13
Papaverine, intravenous injection   53
Para-articular heterotopic ossification   22
Paraesthesiae
   during flexion-extension radiographs   20
Paramedics   12
Paraplegia
   conversion to tetraplegia   51
   fertility   53
   functional electrical stimulation   55
   gait expectations   39
   independence expected   46
Parasympathetic connections   52
Pars interarticularis   21
Passive movements   18, 23, 36, 40
Patient controlled analgesia system (PCAS)
      51
Pelvic twist   33
Pelvicalyceal system   25
Penile implant/prosthesis   27, 52
Penile stimulation   52
Peptic ulceration   16
Perineal toilet   34
Peripheral nerve regeneration   13
Peritoneal lavage   5
Peroneals   55
Perphenazine   51
Personal assistant   48, 49
Phenol   23
Phenothiazines   52
Phentolamine   27, 28
Phenylpropanolamine   27
Philadelphia collar   19
Phrenic nerve   12
Physiotherapy   12, 36–9
Pillows
   uses   15, 17, 33

Placement, assessment, and counselling teams
      (PACTs)   42, 45
Plantar response   6
Poikilothermia   4, 31, 34
Positioning of unconscious patients   2
Positions of cervical spine   19
Positions of patients
   lateral   2, 4, 31, 36
   lateral decubitus   16
   neutral   2
   prone   2
   semiprone (recovery)   2
   supine   2, 4, 31, 33
Posterior columns   5, 6
Posterior cord syndrome   6
Postural hypotension   19, 37, 38
Postural reduction   15
Posturing   31
Power, loss   2
Prazosin   27, 29
Prescription charges, relief   44
Pressure   33, 34
   counter   33
Pressure areas
   accident and emergency department   31
   checking by patient   46
   nursing care   33
   wheelchair   37
Pressure clinic   23, 46
Pressure sores   4, 17, 34, 47
   indications for surgery   23
   plaster casts   18
   prevention   4, 23, 34, 37, 46, 48, 54
   scalp   15
   treatment   23
Priapism   5
Profiling   19
   bed   19, 31, 37
Prognosis   1, 6, 55
   patient acceptance   30
Prone position in tetraplegia   17
Prone trolley for children   50
Propantheline   25, 27
Proprioception   6, 37, 39
Prostatectomy, transurethral   27
Prostatic obstruction   27
Proteus   24
Psychological factors   30, 48, 54
Pulmonary
   contusion   12
   embolism   17, 22, 55
   infection   12, 18
   oedema   13
Pyelonephritis   26

Quadriceps   55
Quadriplegia   1 See Tetraplegia
Quality of life   42

Radial extensors   54
Radiographs   19
   abdominal   16
   anteroposterior   7, 8, 10
   flexion-extension   20
   lateral   7, 8, 9, 10
   oblique   10
   supine   8
Radiography   2
   for evidence of bony union   19
   for position   19
Radiological investigations
   cervical spine   7–10
   peritoneal cavity   16
   thoracolumbar injuries   11
Radiological signs   9
RAF turning frame   18
Ranitidine   16
Reality training   34
Reciprocating gait orthosis (RGO)   38, 39, 55
Recovery position   2
Recreation   42
Reduction   20, 22
Reflexes   3, 5, 6 See also individual reflexes

Index

nerve supply 5
Regression, psychological 30
Rehabilitation 54
  aim 43
  children 39
  landmarks 30
  physical 37–8
  workshop 42
Relationships 47
  breakdown 48, 49
  changed 30, 43
  fulfilment 53
Relatives *See* Family
Relaxation techniques 51, 52
Renal
  failure 55
  function 25, 26
  ultrasonography 25, 26
Renography 25
Respiration
  diaphragmatic 2, 12
  prone position 2
Respiratory
  complications 12, 34
  depression 51
  failure 55
  function 12
  tract infection 18, 55
Respite care 49
Resuscitation 2, 12, 31
Retropulsion 9
Rhizotomy 52
Rib fractures 10, 12
Road traffic accidents 1
Rollator 39
Rotation 2, 4
Rugby Football Union 56

Sacral anterior nerve root stimulator
  (SARS) 29, 52
Sacral reflex arcs 6
Sacrum
  pressure 23, 33, 37
  segments sparing 6
Sandbags 2, 4, 7, 15, 31
Scalp pressure sores 15
Scoliosis 39, 50
Seager electroejaculation unit 53
Self esteem 40, 42, 43
Self harm 1
Self intermittent catheterisation 25, 26, 34, 47
  fluid balance 33, 34
  optimum requirements 25
Seminal emission 52–53
Sensation, altered 2
Sensory input 34
Sensory loss 29, 30, 34, 37, 39, 53
  and fear 30
  hazards 34
  in syringomyelia 51
Sexual function 27, 52–3
Sexual intercourse 53
Sexuality 35
Shock
  hypovolaemic 3, 13
  neurogenic 13
  spinal 5, 6, 16
Sickness benefit 44
Skin 17, 31, 34, 46
Skull calipers 13
Skull traction 13–5, 18, 19, 20, 21
  aims 13
  force 14, 15, 21
Social
  needs 43–5
  services 48
  workers 41, 48
Spasticity 38
  advantages 22
  factors aggravating 22–3
  treatment 22–3, 54
Sperm count 53
Sphincterotomy, distal urethral 27, 28

Spinal
  alignment 31
  anaesthesia 28
  artery compression 6
  board 4
  bone compression 22
  brace 22
  canal 9, 11
  deformity 2, 5, 22, 50
  fusion 15, 20, 21
  immobiliser 4
  incomplete injury 22
  injury 5
  instability 8, 10, 15, 19, 52
  shock 5, 6, 15, 35
  stability 8, 19
Spinal cord
  cavitation 51
  compression 11
  diameter 13
  necrosis 13
  oedema 12, 55
  stimulation 51, 52
Spinal cord injury
  acute 6
  anatomy 13
  associated injuries 5, 12
  causes of 1
  cervical 3, 34
  completeness of 52, 53
  complications 12–3, 16, 30, 50–6
  diagnosis 5–11
  early management 12–8
  high 3, 33
  incidence in UK 1
  incomplete lesions 6, 22, 39
  initial hospital management 5
  later management 50–6
  level of 52
  low 3, 26
  lumbar 38, 52
  mortality 1, 55
  prevention 56
  prognosis 1, 55
  rising level 36
  sacral 52
  signs and symptoms 2, 3, 5–11
  thoracic, low 38
  thoracic, upper 3, 34
  transection 11
Spinal injuries units
  number in UK 18
  nursing organisation 30
  transfer to 18
  visits by community staff 48, 49
Spinal Injuries Association 45, 49
Spinothalamic tractotomy 52
Spinothalamic tracts 5, 6
Spinous processes: radiography 8
Splinting 2, 4, 13, 40, 54
Spondylitis, ankylosing 9
Spondylosis, cervical 6, 9, 15
Sport 38
Sports injuries 1
Sputum retention 12
Stab injuries 6, 15
Stabilisation 2, 13–5
Stamey colposuspension 28
Standing 38, 55
State benefits 48
Statutory care facilities 49
Statutory sick pay 44
Sternal fractures 10, 22
Steroid use 18
Stockings, antiembolism 17, 19
Stones 26, 28
Straight lifting 32
Stress
  and gastrointestinal ulcers 18
  and pressure sores 34
  and rehabilitation landmarks 30, 43
  of nursing staff 30
Stretcher, "scoop" 4

Stryker frame 17, 18, 31
Suction, pharyngeal 3, 4, 13
Supervision by doctor 7, 10, 20
Support, psychological 30, 31
Suppositories 35
Suprapubic catheterisation 16, 24, 28, 35
  fluid balance in 34
Suprapubic
  compression 27
  "tapping" 27
Suprasacral cord lesions 26, 27, 29
Suxamethonium: risk in use of 13
Sweating 46
Switzerland 18
Swivel walker 39, 50
Sympathetic
  outflow 13, 52
  overactivity 28
  paralysis 3, 4, 13, 19
Syringomyelia, post-traumatic 51

Teardrop fracture 9
Technology, modern 42
Temperature
  impaired response to 4
  raised 34
  sensation 6
  testicular 53
Temporalis muscle function and Cone caliper
  insertion 14
Tendon lengthening 23
Tendon transfer 55
Tenodesis 54
Tenotomy 23
Tetraplegia
  arms 33
  choice of bed 31
  expectation of independence 41, 46, 49
  hand 18, 40, 54
  high 47
  hypothermia 4
  indwelling catheter 28
  low 27
  male fertility 53
  mobility 46, 47
  mortality 1
  pressure relief 37
  respiration 2, 36
  rising level of injury 36
  splinting 40
  transporting 18
  vagal tone 13
  vasomotor responses 4
  ventilation-perfusion mismatch 12
  vomiting 16
Thermal reflector sheets 4
Thigh muscle depth 55
Thoracic spinal cord 13
  blood supply 13
  injuries 3, 13
Thoracolumbar injuries 16, 22, 33
  early management 15
  gait re-education 38
  radiological investigations 10
Thromboembolism: prophylaxis 17, 34
Thumb flexion restoration 54
Tilt table 38
Tiredness 30, 34, 44, 48
Toenails 23, 34
Tomography, computed 8, 11, 51
Tracheostomy 12
Traction *See also* Skull traction
  in cervical radiography 8, 19
  injury in children 9
Transcutaneous aspiration 53
Transcutaneous nerve stimulation 51, 52
Transfer skills 37, 39, 47, 54
Transfer to community 46–9
Transportation 4, 12
Trauma trolley 31
Travel to hospital, relief for 44
Triceps tendon 54
Tricyclic antidepressants 52

Trigeminal nerve 51
Trismus: cone caliper insertion 14
Trochanter, pressure sores 23, 37
Trunk control 37
Turns 2, 32–3

Ultrasound measurement of residual urine
    24, 25, 26
Unconscious patient 2–3
Uncontrolled voids 27
University of Virginia caliper 14
Unstable injuries 3
Upright posture in children 39
Urethral
    closure, incompetent 27
    damage 25, 35
    dilatation 25, 28
    distal sphincter obstruction 27
    distal sphincterotomy 27, 28
    diverticulum 26
Urinary
    catheterisation 16, 24–5, 34, 47
    sepsis: death rate in 1917 24
    sphincter, artificial 29
    stones 16
    tract infection 16, 18, 24, 26, 34, 47
Urine

acidification 26, 47
culture 24, 25
infected 25, 28
leaking 27
residual 24, 25, 26, 29
voiding 27
volume 16, 24
Urography 25, 26
Urological management
    early 24–6
    investigations 25–6
    later 26–9, 48

Vacuum erection aid 53
Vagal reflex 3
Vagal tone 13, 28
Ventilation 20
    artificial 12
    domiciliary 12
Ventilation-perfusion mismatch 12
Vertebrae
    compression fracture 6
    crush fracture 9
    lateral mass fracture 6
    "recoil" position 13
    subluxation 9
Vertebrectomy 22

Vesicoureteric reflux 26, 27
Vibrator to induce seminal emission 52, 53
Videourodynamics 26
Vietnam war 13
Visceral stimulation in autonomic
    dysreflexia 28
Vomiting
    tetraplegia 16
    unconscious patient 2
    unintubated supine patient 4

Walking: functional electrical stimulation 55
Walking aids for children 39, 50
War disablement pension 44
Warfarin 17
Weight gain 47
Wheelchair
    assessment for 41, 46
    children 39
    design 38
    home adaptation 41, 44
    mobilisation into 19, 30, 37
    skills 38
    types 41
Withdrawal, psychological 30
Work See Employment
Wrist extension 54